"If you purchase only one book this year, let it be *Winners' Guide to Pain Relief*. Home physical therapy for musculoskeletal pain often fails or falls short of its goal because the necessary ingredients of proper stretching, proper breathing, body positioning and trigger point release are not in place. This book empowers you to develop a home therapy program that will help you discover and ease the source of some of your pain and improve your muscle function."

Devin Starlanyl, Researcher and Author

"Dr. Hal Blatman's book, *Winners' Guide to Pain Relief* is an excellent and much needed source of information on the origins and treatment of myofacial pain. He takes complex medical information and presents it in an easy to understand format that also incorporates his compassion, humor and uniquely personal approach. Dr. Blatman's book will motivate and inspire you the reader to learn the importance of a self-management plan that includes a variety of techniques and exercises that will help you decrease your musculoskeletal pain."

Lynne Matallana, President and Co-Founder, National Fibromyalgia Association

"Dr. Blatman has succeeded in producing a clear, concise and funny book telling us why we hurt. You will learn the proper care and feeding of your muscles, joints, tendons, and ligaments to relieve and prevent chronic musculoskeletal pain. This is a must have book if you are a treating health care practitioner, avid health nut, athelete or someone in chronic pain. This invaluable resource clearly explains what is essential to treat and prevent one of the most common causes of chronic pain."

Dr. Rick Marinelli, Naturopathic Physician

"Dr. Blatman has produced an incredible work! Nowhere in my 20 plus years as a therapist and teacher have I seen a popular book so well written and illustrated that most anyone can pick it up, understand the concepts, and get pain relief right now! I regularly receive calls from all over the country asking what people can do for themselves. This book is the answer to that question."

Richard Finn, Director of Pittsburgh School of Pain Management

"Dr. Blatman knows muscles! His book provides you with techniques to manage your muscles everyday. If you have myofascial pain symptoms, you will find the excellent illustrations and easy to follow instructions most helpful in guiding you (and your muscles) to a successful self-treatment program. I enjoyed this book and recommend it for those with myofascial pain syndrome."

Mark J. Pellegrino, MD, Author and Expert on Fibromyalgia

"Hal Blatman is a master of the art of pain management. For those of you who are tired of medication side effects, or who are simply tired of being in pain, this book will do a spectacular job of teaching you, in a simple and easy to understand way, what you can do yourself to get pain free now! A must read!"

Jacob Teitelbaum MD, Author of *Pain Free 1-2-3!*

The Art of Body Maintainence:
Winners' Guide To
PAIN
RELIEF

By
Hal Blatman, MD
Brad Ekvall, BFA

Danua Press, LLC

Illustrations and graphic design by Brad Ekvall
Cover design by Brad Ekvall

Printed and bound in the United States of America by CJK

Published by:
    Danua Press, L.L.C.
    10653 Techwoods Circle
    Suite 101
    Cincinnati, OH   45242

Telephone: 513-956-3200
Fax: 513-956-3206
e-mail: drblatman@blatmanpainclinic.com
Web: blatmanpainclinic.com
                     winoverpain.com

ISBN: 9780972968003
Library of Congress Control Number: 2006900360

1 1-06

TABLE of CONTENTS

ACKNOWLEDGMENTS

A very special thanks goes to Mary Gilbert for her many hours reviewing earlier versions of this book and for her patience as she taught me to write. Her husband Jay also deserves great appreciation for his tolerance as Mary gave so freely of her time in helping us.

Thanks to my parents Don and Lois for teaching me to believe in myself. Lois was alive and supportive when I began writing and, in addition to his encouragement throughout the years, Don has reviewed and provided his input on several versions of this book.

I thank my wife Nancy whose encouragement, patience, love, and support I count on every day. Our children Joshua and Daniel have also taught me much throughout my professional career.

Sadly, Brad's father Ray is also not here to see this book published. For the many hours he spent meticulously pouring over the early draft and for his fresh perspective on the final version, we are most grateful.

I have had many mentors while learning about myofascial pain and the techniques described in this book. Among them is Dr. Larry Funt who organized the first courses I attended, allowing me to learn directly from Dr. Janet Travell. In addition to teaching me about myofascial pain, injection techniques, and the importance of nutritional supplementation, Dr. Travell helped open my senses to the great variety of possibilities in helping people in their paths of healing from pain. Since then, my clinic staff has helped develop our patient home care program that is described in this book. Lastly, my most important teachers have been my patients. They have helped develop and validate this work over the many years I have been in practice.

FOREWORD

This book is one of the most important tools available to improve your function and the quality of your life. Now, for the first time, a physician specializing in myofascial pain treatment has written a book for you.

This book is a maintenance manual for the
human musculoskeletal system.
If you have a musculoskeletal system, you need
this book!

No matter what body work you have had done *to you*, the work *you do for yourself* is more important. Your body-worker is with you for only a short time. *You* are the one who lives in your body all the time.

Through the diagrams skillfully illustrated by Brad Ekvall B.F.A., you will see various techniques to treat yourself as your own "personal in-home massage therapist." You will learn when and how to stretch in a healthy manner, even if you are elderly or have a coexisting condition such as fibromyalgia syndrome. As you read, you will learn the proper breathing techniques with each exercise from the same person who taught me. We all breathe and we all move—but we need to learn to do these more effectively.

Dr. Hal Blatman was taught directly by the late Dr. Janet Travell, one of the founders of myofascial medicine and treatment. He was also invited to teach with her...a very impressive opportunity.

When I started writing books and working long hours, I spent a week with Dr. Blatman to take a layer off my pain and increase my function. In the morning, Dr. Blatman used his considerable Myofascial Trigger Point (TrP) injection skills and his myo-therapy team went to work on some of my worst TrPs. They taught me several stretches and introduced me to the "ball work" that is featured in this book.

His skill in pain management was so effective, that I was able to get treatment in the morning, work all afternoon, and then often speak to local support groups in the evening without stress to my body and mind—in spite of severe fibromyalgia and chronic myofascial pain.

Last year I wrote a 400-page text, was lead researcher on a clinical study, and took part in two other medical journal papers—and every day I did my stretches and ball work that I learned from the one week I spent with Dr. Blatman.

At last, with this manual, I can reinforce my training and understand my pain patterns in more depth. It is my great pleasure to invite you to do likewise.

Devin J. Starlanyl

Author of:

Fibromyalgia and Myofascial Pain: A Survival Manual, with Mary Ellen Copeland and Christopher R. Brown, 2001

The Fibromyalgia Advocate, 1998

Chronic Myofascial Pain Syndrome: A Guide to the Trigger Points video 1997
Informational website http://www.sover.net/~devstar

Worlds of Power, Lines of Light*, 1999 (FMS and CMP-related science fiction)*

MY JOURNEY
by Hal Blatman

How I Got Started

My medical education was solidly based in conventional medicine. I received my MD degree from The Medical College of Pennsylvania, and started my residency training in Orthopedic Surgery. This training was excellent, and I was fascinated by what I was able to learn about the human body.

I was also impressed by the people with chronic pain conditions who did not seem to be helped by the standard types of treatment. Basic treatments included physical therapy, antiinflammatory medication, injections of cortisone, and surgery. Despite my best efforts, patients returned to the clinic on a monthly basis to remind me that their knees still hurt, their backs hurt, and they still had the headaches that started with their neck injuries.

A couple of years later, I left the orthopedic surgery program and was working in a small clinic setting. People in pain from various musculoskeletal injuries came for care, as well as many with various types of headaches. One day in the early 1980's, a dentist came to visit with me in the clinic. He taught me about headaches, myofascial pain, and TMJ syndrome. Most of what he discussed was totally new to me, and with this new information I began to examine people with head and neck pain much differently. I found that headaches were almost always associated with tender knots in the muscles of the jaw, neck, and upper shoulders.

My next milestone in learning occurred several years later when I was called upon to examine a woman with severe lower abdominal and pelvic pain. Her lower abdomen was extremely tender, so much so that the medical term "rebound tenderness" applied. Paradoxically, there was nothing in her medical history or basic evaluation that supported the notion of her having a pelvic infection. Instead of transporting her to a local hospital for further evaluation, I offered to stretch out the muscles in her abdomen first. Several days before, my friend and medical director had given me an article on myofascial pain written by Dr. Janet Travell. The patient agreed to my offer, and I stretched the muscles of her abdomen according to the directions in the article.

Within a few minutes, and much to my amazement, she was pain free and her abdominal tenderness had disappeared. During the next few weeks, I read the rest of the article that Dr. Travell had written. I soon realized that what my friend taught me about myofascial head and neck pain applied to muscles throughout the entire body.

After this point, my clinical work began to take on a new direction. I was eager to evaluate patients with pain problems, and I began to read and teach myself about myofascial pain. Trigger point injections and vapocoolant spray and stretch became more important and useful in my practice than anti-inflammatory medications.

In 1988, after finishing a residency training program in Occupational and Environmental medicine, I started the first medical practice in my area of the country that was focused on treating people with myofascial pain disorders. As this practice grew, it evolved into treating people with sports injury pain and people with chronic pain and fibromyalgia syndrome. During my early years of practice, I was also very fortunate to have the opportunity to study and learn from Dr. Travell. She answered so many of my questions and was a wonderful teacher.

Changes in Medical Thinking and Diagnosis

The more I learned about myofascial pain, the more I realized the prevalence of the condition. Almost all of the pain patients I examined had tender and active myofascial trigger points in their muscles that caused or contributed to their pain. I began to question the meaning of several conventional diagnostic terms, including:

Tendonitis referred to inflammation caused by overuse of the muscle.

Migraine headache was supposed to come from blood vessel changes near the brain, and tension headache was supposed to come from tension and stress.

Pleurisy referred to pain coming from inflammation in the tissue lining the outside of the lung and the inside of the chest wall.

Carpal tunnel syndrome was thought to be caused by inflammation and swelling of the wrist/forearm tendons that then squished the median nerve that also passes through the wrist.

Growing pains were the mysteriously mild to severe pains that occurred in otherwise normal and active children that did not seem to be related to injury and usually went away by themselves.

Phantom limb pain was a mysterious pain that felt like it came from legs or arms that had been amputated.

As I questioned the origin of each of these disorders, I noticed that they often responded to treatment directed towards the myofascial system of the body. Tendonitis and bursitis patients always had trigger points. Migraine headache was almost always related to trigger points in jaw, neck, shoulder, and upper back muscles. Pleurisy often resolved with treatment of trigger points under the arms. Carpal tunnel syndrome responded to stretching of fascia. Growing pains were immediately resolved by trigger point injection.

And phantom limb pain was largely caused by muscles that remained in the body after amputation surgery. Indeed, "myofascial medicine" was often more effective and safer than anti-inflammatory medications and traditional therapy choices.

During the next several years, my experience grew in the art of physical examination, as did my desire to share this information with patients and colleagues. Thus, I sat down to write this book more than 13 years ago.

Brad joined me a few years later. We spent many hours discussing the concepts I wanted to communicate and the drawings that ultimately came to relate the information so effectively.

As you read through this book, my thoughts regarding each of these conditions is further explained. I hope that you too will find that these conditions usually respond to the techniques of stretching and massage that are illustrated here.

introduction

introduction

HOW THIS BOOK CAN HELP

This book takes the mystery out of pain, teaching you where pain comes from and how you can make it go away. As a result, you will have more control over acute pain as well as chronic pain and the pain flares that come after "doing too much."

Conventional medical training teaches that pain comes from:

inflammation

pinched nerves

herniated discs

depression

it's in your head

The **traditional medical model** treats pain with surgery, various types of injection blocks, psychology, and medication:

anti-inflammatory

opioid

antidepressant

anti-seizure

sleep

Alternative medicine treatments include:

massage

reflexology

chiropractic

acupuncture

biofeedback

relaxation

While all these methods can be helpful and each has a place in pain management, none take the mystery out of pain treatment and give people the power to understand their pain and treat themselves. As a result, people continue to be dependent on their doctors, and their pain typically worsens between treatments as they struggle to make overall progress.

A *pain pattern* is the location of pain in the body. The *quality* of pain is what the pain feels like such as aching, cramping, knife-like, or numbness and tingling. We are taught that the quality and location of a pain pattern indicate different causes for the pain. Examples include thinking that numbness is caused by a nerve injury, back pain is caused by arthritis, or neck stiffness is caused by a pinched nerve. While these examples can certainly be true, it is also true that these qualities of pain can all be caused by muscle. Indeed, even very severe and sharp pain can be caused by muscle. Pain that comes from muscle is called **myofascial pain**.

The term "**myofascial**" is derived from the words "**myo**" which means muscle, and "**fascia**" which is the connective tissue that covers and intertwines with muscle. Muscle injuries, including those from sudden strain, repetitive strain, and trauma cause knots to form in the muscle and fascia tissue. These knots are called myofascial trigger points (TrPs). With practice, they can be felt in the muscles near the location of almost any pain pattern. **Myofascial pain** is the pain that is generated by these knots. Physiologically, these knots (trigger points) are hyperactive focal areas of irritability in muscle or its associated fascia.

Most of the pain in the body is indeed myofascial pain. Everything from plantar fascitis to migraine headache can be treated with the methods described in this book. The degree of success will vary from one person to another, but most pain patterns have a myofascial component, and the techniques described in this book will be helpful.

The purpose of this book is to instruct you to understand and self-treat myofascial pain symptoms from head to toe. It can be used by itself or in conjunction with other healing techniques such as chiropractic, massage therapy, or acupuncture. When used in conjunction with other treatment, you become a more active participant in your own healing process. This will result in greater and faster improvement.

With this different understanding about the cause of pain, symptoms that are usually called "*arthritis, tendonitis, bursitis, pinched nerve, herniated disc,* and *pain from depression*" may become more treatable.

In addition to understanding and treating pain, this book teaches about body maintenance. Just as we need to maintain our automobiles, we need to maintain our bodies. Proper maintenance with massage and stretching promotes greater flexibility and improved athletic performance.

Pain that does not seem to respond to conventional medical treatment may well respond to the techniques described in this book.

Myofascial pain syndrome is an all too common and very unsettling condition that often affects people with a history of musculoskeletal injury. It can be diagnosed in association with different types of injury. Most commonly myofascial pain is diagnosed in people who are still suffering several years after an apparent "strain" injury. Common examples include *chronic lower back pain, neck pain, and headache.* Myofascial pain is also the predominant problem in people with pain from *repetitive motion injuries.* Commonly diagnosed conditions such as *tennis elbow* and *bursitis* have a significant myofascial component. Lastly, much of the pain caused by acute injuries to muscle is also myofascial in origin. Common acute injuries include conditions diagnosed as muscular

Myofascial Pain is part of almost any chronic pain condition.

tears (i.e. calf and hamstring). In many people, these injuries cause some element of disability and a tendency towards re-injury and exacerbation of pain with certain physical activities. Examples include professional athletes with recurrent injuries.

Indeed, myofascial pain *should be considered part of almost any chronic pain condition.*

HOW TO USE THIS BOOK

The **Introduction** explains basic concepts regarding myofascial pain syndrome. A summary of standard medical education for the diagnosis and treatment of pain is presented, along with a basic description of the theory of myofascial pain syndrome.

The **Map Chapter** illustrates locations of pain symptoms and which muscles are likely to be causing a particular pain pattern. Usually there is more than one muscle responsible for causing any pain pattern. To use this section, first think of which regions of your body are involved in your pain pattern. Then compare the location of your pain symptoms with the pain diagrams in this section. Make note of which muscles cause pain patterns that match the location of any part of your pain. Trigger point locations are marked in the diagrams by the "angry face" icons and "lightning bolts" pointing to the body locations. Pain patterns are illustrated by clusters of smaller "angry face" icons.

Next, the **Ball Massage Chapter** illustrates how to massage each of these muscles using an ordinary ball about the size of a tennis ball. When these techniques are performed, the body responds much like it will to acupressure and massage therapy. Acupressure is treatment of trigger points with pressure that physically makes them smaller. Smaller trigger points generate less pain. Massage therapy is beneficial in part because toxins are massaged or squeezed out of the muscles, leaving more room for fresh blood and nutrients. Using the ball helps the muscles "breathe" better.

The **Stretching Chapter** is divided into two sections. **Part 1**, *General Principles of Stretching*, discusses important ideas, methods, and goals of stretching. The real "cure" for myofascial pain is stretching the involved muscles to their normal length. Aggressive stretching can cause an increase in pain, and proper technique will facilitate the healing process and body maintenance for the activities that we enjoy in life.

Be sure to read the General Principles of Stretching Section before starting to do stretching exercises.

It is important to work repetitively with the breathing and relaxation techniques described. Do not be discouraged if you do not "get it" on the first try. Relaxation is the most important key to stretching, and sometimes the hardest thing to do is "to do nothing" and relax. With practice your ability to relax into deeper and deeper levels will improve and the results of your efforts will be more noticeable.

Part 2, *Stretching Positions*, illustrates body positioning and directions for movement in performing stretching exercises. Each muscle technique is illustrated and described in detail. The stretching chapter is placed after the ball chapter to emphasize the importance of using the ball before stretching. This is certainly not necessary, but in general, it is almost always easier to stretch a muscle after it has been massaged with the ball.

The **Picture Index** allows for quickly locating the pages that teach ball massage and stretching techniques for any listed pain pattern.

Traditional Medical Theories for Chronic Pain

The medical profession teaches several theories, or models, to explain pain and chronic pain. Understanding what doctors are taught may help you understand your diagnosis better. It may also help you understand why you have more than one diagnosis for your pain condition.

One theory is the **"inflammation" model**. This model includes diagnoses such as tendonitis, bursitis, and arthritis. Inflammation can certainly cause pain, however, it is often not the only cause of pain in the area of symptoms.

Doctors often order x-ray studies of joints in the areas of pain symptoms. If there is evidence of degenerative change, the diagnosis is arthritis. We are all taught that arthritis comes with age, and that it causes pain. When the doctor tells us that we have a "touch of arthritis," we quickly accept the diagnosis as a reasonable cause of our pain. As an orthopedic resident I had the opportunity to examine patients before their total hip surgeries. Some had good range of motion, normal joint space on x-ray, and tremendous pain in their hip joints. Others had a very limited range of motion, no pain, and bone on bone x-ray findings. The **x-rays** correlated with the patients' range of motion, but they **did not correlate with the degree of pain** symptoms.

Another hypothesis is called the **"pinched nerve/herniated disc" model**. Many people suffer with numbness, tingling, and burning pain that radiates into an arm or leg. Physicians are taught that this pain comes from a pinching injury to a nerve, closer to the spinal cord than the location of the symptoms. MRI scans and EMG testing are done in an effort to look for an injured disc and the nerve being pinched. In many people, however, the MRI scans and EMG tests are normal in the face of persistent symptoms. Even when there is evidence of a herniated disc, surgery may not provide relief or improvement. Then, when pain worsens after surgery, the physician may suggest that "scar tissue" from the surgery is the reason for continued symptoms. Sometimes when pain continues after good medical or surgical treatment, it is even thought that these people are malingering (faking their pain for some other goal i.e. a legal settlement or an "off-work" note).

A few years ago a medical study examined middle aged men who never had low back pain or low back injury. Each of these men underwent a lumbar spine scan study, and approximately 30 percent of them had at least one herniated lumbar disc. The study demonstrated that herniated discs do not always cause pain symptoms!

The **"neurogenic or neuralgia" model** explains tingling and burning pain when no evidence can be found for a pinched nerve. Indeed, sometimes nerves not only transmit pain signals, but they also generate pain signals. When this happens, the perceived pain is often much greater than what would be expected from the original injury. One example of this kind of diagnosis is "occipital neuralgia" causing headache pain. Sometimes this is proven by injecting local anesthetic (i.e. Novocaine) to make the nerve numb and relieve the headache. If the pain persists after a successful injection, an effort may be made to kill the nerve with electricity, cold, radio waves, or injection of toxic chemicals into the area. Even when these techniques are successful, pain symptoms may return within a few years.

When these theories cannot be reasonably applied, there are psychological reasons for continued pain that are considered. One example is the **"depressed middle aged woman" model** for pain. This theory is tragic beyond words. Many women with significant and treatable pain are "blown-off" in this manner. Because they are not taken seriously, they become more depressed and their symptoms magnify. It is true that many people with chronic pain are women and many of these women are middle aged and suffer from some form of depression. Doctors have been taught that the depression comes first and thereby causes the pain condition. The truth, however, is that chronic pain by itself can cause depression. This occurs because pain sensations from trigger points travel by nerve fibers of the sympathetic nervous system and bombard the brain's mood center. When you get depressed on a bad pain day, *your body can do it to your head*, even if your childhood was normal and your life is perfect.

Another theory is the **"imaginary pain" model**. If medical testing can not find the cause for the pain, and the patient still thinks the pain exists, then the pain must all be in the person's head. The treatment under this diagnosis will most likely be an inpatient *"learn how to live with the pain"* treatment program, or referral to a psychiatrist.

14

Multidisciplinary pain centers teach people how to *"live with their pain."* This treatment may indeed help people who could not be helped in any other manner. Sometimes, however, patients are also sent to these centers for "detox." To this end, these centers have been used to provide society with an avenue to ease its conscience regarding humanitarian values and the use of narcotic pain medication. Physicians and the general public are taught that narcotic medication is addictive and that chronic use is detrimental and dangerous. As a result, sometimes people are referred to these programs so their pain medication can be discontinued in a hospital environment. These people are then discharged from the center with little or no pain medication. This causes untold and unnecessary suffering.

Many people with genuine pain conditions can be given partial pain relief and an improved level of functioning if they are provided with appropriate dosing of narcotic medication.

Unfortunately, these theories and models are seriously incomplete and do not adequately apply to a majority of chronic pain patients. As a result,

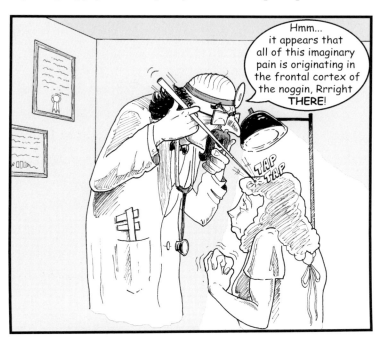

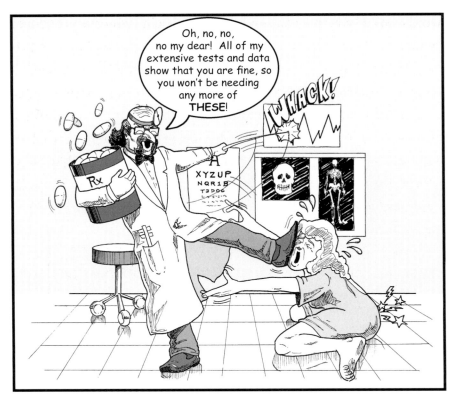

when a person with chronic pain goes to the doctor for treatment, what the person has may not fit what the doctor has been taught.

Myofascial Pain Model for Chronic Pain

There is another theory that helps explain much of chronic pain in a more constructive and productive manner. The **"myofascial pain" model** is more constructive because it gives people hope and a chance to lessen or get rid of their pain. Altogether, it is more productive because treatment in accordance with this model usually provides significant restoration of function and relief from pain. I have found that very few medical training programs include teaching about this model. The condition is underdiagnosed, and rarely treated optimally according to the protocols described by those who pioneered the field since the 1940's.

As stated previously (page 9) the term **"myofascial"** is derived from the words "**myo**" which means muscle, and "**fascia**" which is the connective tissue that covers and intertwines with muscle. **Myofascial pain** is the pain that is generated by hyperactive focal areas of irritability in muscle or its associated fascia that are called *myofascial trigger points*. A trained examiner can usually detect these trigger points with palpation. They feel like knots in the muscle, and they are usually located within a taught, ropy band of muscle. By what these knots feel like, a skilled examiner can often tell where a person hurts, even without being shown. The diagnosis of myofascial pain is determined mostly by physical examination, and seldom by medical testing.

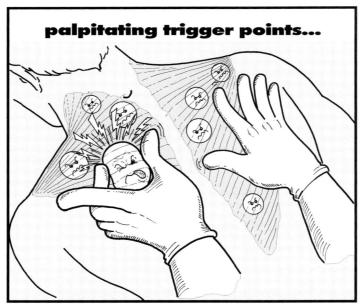

Trigger points are described in three ways: *active*, *latent*, and *satellite*.

An **active trigger point** typically causes pain at rest and more pain when the muscle is used. Active trigger points typically refer pain, numbness, tingling, or burning to other areas of the body.

Latent trigger points do not usually cause pain that a person is conscious of; however, they cause weakness and restriction of motion on an indefinite basis. There is usually no evidence of atrophy or muscle wasting associated with the weakness. Latent trigger points persist for many years after an injury. They may also become more active with overuse of the muscle, chilling, or leaving the muscle in a shortened position for a prolonged period of time. A common example of activation of latent trigger points is the phenomenon known as a "stiff neck." This may occur when latent trigger points in neck and upper shoulder musculature activate during the night, causing extreme neck pain and stiffness the next morning.

Satellite trigger points develop in the zone of referred pain from another trigger point. For example, if a neck muscle trigger point refers

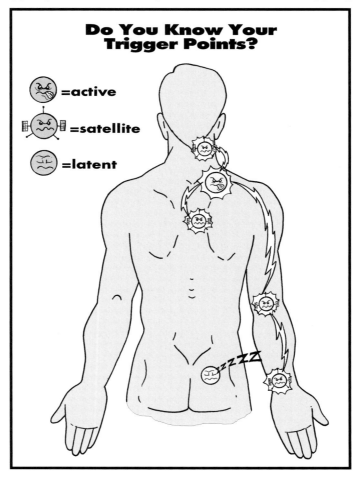

pain into the arm and forearm long enough, the musculature of the arm and forearm will develop trigger points even in the absence of direct trauma to the area. These satellite trigger points typically have the same characteristics as other active trigger points in that they generate pain, restrict motion, and cause weakness without atrophy. Consequently, the concept of measuring limb circumference in evaluating reported weakness in a person with chronic pain may be basically flawed.

Myofascial trigger points may generate different qualities of pain. The pain can be knife-like and stabbing, dull and achy, burning, or numb and tingly.

Typical examples of myofascial pain syndromes include headaches that are often diagnosed as tension, sinus, or migraine. Neck pain that radiates into the arm and forearm, as well as lower back pain that radiates into the thigh and leg are often myofascial in origin. When a person has radiation of burning pain, numbness, and tingling into an extremity, and when they have normal MRI scans and normal EMG studies, then the symptoms are almost always myofascial pain. These symptoms will usually improve and often resolve with treatment directed towards the myofascial component of the pain pattern.

PERPETUATING FACTORS FOR MYOFASCIAL PAIN SYNDROME

There are several factors that perpetuate myofascial pain and increase the likelihood that a pain pattern will progress to involve more of the body and subsequently, cause depression and sleep disturbance problems.

Perpetuating factors include:
- *structural inadequacies* (i.e. one leg shorter than the other)
- *nutritional inadequacies* (especially vitamin C, various B complex vitamins, magnesium)
- *ergonomic factors* (activities of daily living and work that physically

aggravate the involved muscles)
- *metabolic conditions* (hypothyroidism)
- *psychological problems* (depression, anxiety, anger)
- *nutrition (*foods that perpetuate myofascial pain)

Nutritional perpetuating factors include poisons such as aspartame and hydrogenated oil, processed food such as sugar and white flour, and caffeine.

TREATMENT OF MYOFASCIAL PAIN TO DIMINISH CHRONIC PAIN

In treating chronic myofascial pain, all of these perpetuating factors must be addressed. For most people, this will make improvement easier and quicker. For others, correction of perpetuating factors will make treatment possible.

Structural inadequacies such as a short leg may be addressed with a simple heel lift inside a shoe. Others will need a more complex orthosis. Nutritional inadequacies may be addressed by making better food choices, and taking vitamins and other nutritional supplements. Correction of ergonomic factors may mean using a headset with the phone and changing the position of office equipment. Metabolic conditions can often be diagnosed by medical testing and corrected with medication. Psychological problems may be helped with many techniques, including various forms of therapy, biofeedback, and medication.

Body work is another important part of myofascial pain treatment. The goal of this work is to make trigger points less active and thereby lessen the pain that they cause. Stretch is often a key to success with this work. This is accomplished with the help of **five tools**:

rubber ball

repetition of stretching

vapocoolant spray (cold spray *that helps unlock muscle*)

hands-on massage/myotherapy
trigger point injections

The **rubber ball** is used to apply pressure to the trigger points and also to do massage. Compressing a trigger point with pressure from the ball will be uncomfortable and can easily be painful. It is important to relax with the

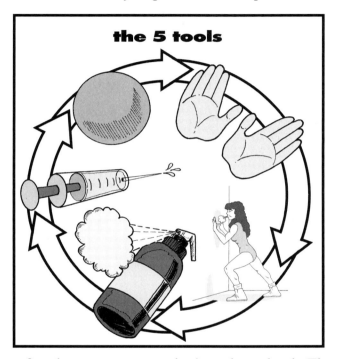

the 5 tools

level of discomfort that you cause, so don't push too hard. The discomfort you can relax with is called a "good hurt." If you do push too hard, your muscle may tighten even more or you may bruise. This is not likely to cause serious damage, but will cause more soreness. In general, maintaining pressure on a trigger point will cause the trigger point to become smaller and less active. The trigger point will subsequently generate less pain and the muscle will stretch further and more easily. The ball can also be used for self-massage by rolling it over areas of the body.

Repetitive stretching helps to restore the involved musculature to its normal and healthy resting length. Some people may need to stretch 10 to

15 times per day to succeed in treatment. The goal of stretching is to prevent tightening of the muscles from the stress of the day's activities. Interestingly, we have discovered that how far you stretch **DOES NOT COUNT.** Distance is not worth the effort! Do your stretches very slowly, do not stretch into pain, and **do not pull on your body**. If the muscles are "stuck," they need to be loosened with other tools. One such tool is the **rubber ball** which is discussed previously. It is mentioned first to emphasize that you will improve faster and have an easier time with stretching if you use the ball for a few minutes first.

Hands-on massage (done by yourself or with the help of another) is an alternative to the ball. Both hands-on and ball-massage techniques will loosen muscles and help them to stretch further. These techniques will also move toxins out of the muscles and encourage blood flow and cellular nutrition.

Another tool is **vapo-coolant spray** such as Fluori-methane or Ethyl Chloride. These sprays block reflex pain and spasm during stretching, and allow the muscle to stretch without pain. This technique may be done by the physical therapist, and you can usually be taught how to use this yourself. The spray usually requires a prescription and can be purchased at the pharmacy.

The most powerful tool for inactivating trigger points is a **trigger point injection**. The particular agent injected is of little importance and cortisone (an anti-inflammatory medication) is rarely necessary. During the procedure, the muscle will almost always twitch and reproduce its referral pain pattern.

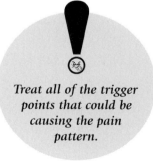

Treat all of the trigger points that could be causing the pain pattern.

Injecting a little novocaine (a local anesthetic and painkiller) can be very helpful. After the trigger point is inactivated, the muscle must be stretched to its more normal length. All of the musculature involved in the pain pattern must also be stretched at the time of the office visit. Remember, the stretch is the "cure," and the injection is merely the tool that allows the stretch to happen. Unfortunately, this protocol is difficult to learn, time consuming, and thus rarely followed in practice.

When myofascial pain conditions are treated in this manner, the pain patterns evolve backwards in time and eventually resolve or reach a plateau of improvement. This can take 6 to 12 months in people with chronic conditions. Occasionally people will continue to steadily improve during the course of two years of treatment. This length of time needed depends upon the severity and duration of the pain condition. While it is easier to treat people sooner after an injury, at least some degree of improvement can be expected even when the injury is 15–20 years old.

While other physical therapy modalities such as ultrasound, electric stim and hot packs are professed to be helpful, my experience is that they usually provide little or no significant improvement in chronic myofascial pain beyond some temporary relief.

INTRODUCTION TO FIBROMYALGIA SYNDROME

Fibromyalgia is the name we give to the condition where several body systems are not working well, and there are symptoms in many of them. In addition to pain, people with fibromyalgia often experience intestinal abnormalities, mentation difficulties, thyroid and other endocrine imbalance, and fatigue. There are several books available that teach about fibromyalgia, and some of the best are written by Dr. Devin Starlanyl.

Fibromyalgia syndrome may coexist with myofascial pain, but the two conditions are not the same. While I have seen people with myofascial pain and no fibromyalgia, I have never seen people with fibromyalgia and no myofascial pain. **Virtually all people with fibromyalgia have myofascial pain** causing a major portion of their pain symptoms.

In most people, myofascial pain involves a small area of the body and responds to treatment directed towards a small "ensemble" of trigger points.

People with fibromyalgia are usually dealing with an "orchestra" of trigger points scattered throughout their bodies.

Coexisting fibromyalgia may complicate the treatment for myofascial pain. In a general way, people with fibromyalgia are more fragile. People with both conditions must follow the guidelines suggested in this book, and be very careful to avoid stretching into pain. Additionally, using the ball will massage toxins from the muscles into the blood stream. These must then be removed through lymph, kidneys, intestines, and skin. Drinking extra water is very important. More fragile people should start very slowly, perhaps using the ball only once each day and on a smaller less painful part of the body. Too many of these toxins in the blood stream can cause flu-like symptoms, including nausea, aches and pains, vomiting, and diarrhea.

People with fibromyalgia might also consider starting with a softer ball, such as a racket ball or a soft rubber ball from the toy store. Another way to soften the pressure of the ball is to wear a sweatshirt or other similar "cushion" clothing.

GENERAL INSTRUCTIONS FOR EVERYONE

In this order, each person's morning routine should include:
ball--shower--stretch.

The most important body work of the day is what you do first thing in the morning. This is also the time of day when it is most difficult to move and stretch. It is always easier to stretch if the ball and moist heat are used first. Be gentle at first, and only "dust" the muscles with the ball. Do not roll over the same part of a muscle more than once or twice until your body is used to the work.

The second most important body work of the day is in the evening before bed. At first, do this soon after dinner so there is time to drink water and pass it before going to bed. Later, you may find that you sleep better if you use the ball close to bedtime. It is easy to understand that relaxing the mind causes relaxation of the muscles. What is not so obvious is that relaxing the muscles will help relaxation of the mind.

After a week or so, it will be possible to use the ball and stretch five to seven brief times per day. Remember to be gentle, and that ten one's still make a ten.

At some point, you will discover the relief that comes from putting the ball on one particular knot and just leaning on it for a few minutes. This direct compression of a trigger point will help promote its release. You will usually get more results from your effort if you stretch right afterwards.

SPECIAL CONSIDERATIONS

Perhaps your doctor or therapist has advised you that stretching is not right for you. It could be that they do not understand what you mean by stretching (as instructed in this book), or it could mean that they have concern that this stretching could delay your recovery or be harmful. In either case, it is likely that gently using the ball techniques will be safe. These techniques alone may be very helpful in reducing pain and speeding recovery.

ANATOMIC LOCATION OF TRIGGER POINTS

Trigger points can be located basically in three areas of any muscle: at the origin, insertion, and belly of the muscle. The origin and insertion are the musculotendinous attachments where the muscles hook into the bone at either end. The muscle belly is everything in between.

You will not be able to use the ball techniques on the trigger points in the muscle origin or insertion. These areas are best treated with injection techniques. They may respond favorably to massage with your thumbs or fingers, but they are too close to bone and the ball is generally going to be too rough. Most of your work should be in the area of the muscle belly. It is in this area where you can be the most help to your body. Using the ball here will promote detoxification and also massage the largest and usually the most active trigger points. It is not always necessary to directly treat the origin and insertion areas.

SYMPATHETIC NERVOUS SYSTEM

The human nervous system has a section that runs many bodily functions automatically. The part of the nervous system that controls the automatic "fight or flight" response is called the sympathetic nervous system. Pain from myofascial trigger points is transmitted to the brain by fibers of the sympathetic nervous system. In addition, this part of the nervous system innervates (talks to) all of the trigger points in the muscles.

This connection is what causes mental tension to result in more muscle tension and pain. In a similar fashion, anxiety also causes more muscle tightening and pain. It follows then, that mental relaxation is key to allowing muscles to soften and stretch. Pay special attention to learning the breathing techniques that are described in **Part 1** of the **Stretching Chapter**.

TYPES OF INJURY

Muscles can be injured by tearing, straining, bruising, and repetitively using the muscle. When muscles are torn, a defect can usually be felt through the skin. Sometimes this type of injury will require a surgical repair. Some of the pain will come from the torn tissue, some from the bleeding and bruising, and some from the trigger points in the tight areas of the muscle.

Straining involves making the muscle lift or move something that is too heavy. There may be microscopic tears in the muscle that lead to bruising. In addition, there are always trigger points in the injured muscle, and these generate most of the pain. This is what happens most of the time when someone's "back goes out" from doing physical activity. Sometimes this activity is a heavy lift, and other times it is just moving the "wrong way" to pick up a Kleenex.

Hitting the muscle causes a contusion or bruise. Often there is bleeding and a bruise that becomes evident during the next few days. Trigger points may form in the area of the bruise, and these may continue to cause pain long after the injury is healed.

Repetitive strain sometimes causes inflammation of the tendons that attach the muscle to bone. It always causes formation and aggravation of trigger points. Examples of this type of injury include Golfer's elbow (see page 174) and Tennis elbow (see page 183).

WHY DO TOXINS BUILD UP IN MUSCLE TISSUE?

Muscles use or burn energy. To do this, they bring in nutrients and send out exhaust, much like an automobile engine. Blood flow carries in nutrients and also carries out most of the exhaust.

Tight bands and knots are areas of the muscle that are using extra energy to stay contracted. Unfortunately, the pressure from contraction prevents extra blood from getting into these areas of tightness. This keeps the muscles from getting enough extra energy, and also prevents adequate washout of the exhaust products (i.e. lactic acid). Examples of this process include sitting in one position too long (for lower back muscles) and driving an automobile (for upper shoulder muscles).

SUGGESTED READING

Dr. Janet Travell wrote scientific articles in the medical literature about myofascial pain since the 1940's. She was President Kennedy's physician, especially with regard to his back pain. One of the best references on the subject of myofascial pain is a two-volume medical text written by Dr. Janet Travell and Dr. David Simons titled: *Myofascial Pain and Dysfunction, The Trigger Point Manual*. Volumes I and II were published by the Williams and Wilkins company in 1983 and 1993 respectively. A newer version of volume one was published in 1999. A *Cliff Notes* version is a monograph written by Dr. Simons titled: *Myofascial Pain Due To Trigger Points*. It may be available from the

Gebauer Company located in Cleveland, Ohio (www.gebauerco.com). This company also makes the vapo-coolant sprays.

Conclusion

The most commonly used methods for treating chronic pain are based on medical theories that do not always work well. Chronic pain patients need physicians and therapists who are more thoroughly trained in treating people based upon the myofascial model of pain. By using this treatment, many more injured people will be able to optimize and reintegrate their normal life routine.

map
chapter

map

USING THIS CHAPTER

The first step in understanding and working on a particular area of pain in the body is to learn where the pain can come from and which muscles need to be treated. Pain is rarely coming from just one muscle. Within hours of an injury, there are usually several muscles involved in any particular pain pattern.

In this section of the book, major locations of body pain are discussed and diagrammed. The locations of muscle groups are shown in the *muscle diagram*. Myofascial trigger points and their pain patterns are shown in the *TrP pain diagram*.

Refer to the pages diagramming the location of pain symptoms and study the trigger point locations that can cause pain in the problem areas. Usually there will be trigger points in more than one muscle that can refer pain to a particular area of the body. Study the diagrams in each body section (i.e. hip, thigh, and calf sections for leg pain) to learn where these muscles and trigger points are most likely located.

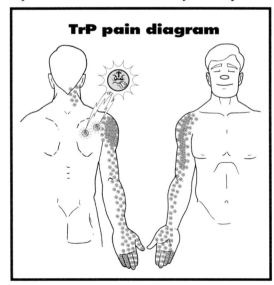

TrP pain diagram

Then turn to the section of the book that describes how to use the rubber ball for massaging these particular muscles and trigger point areas. Start to use the ball for short periods of time (as short as 30 seconds, occasionally several minutes), several times each day. Drink lots of water, as the toxins that you push out of the muscles can make you feel very sick if your kidneys do not flush them out of your

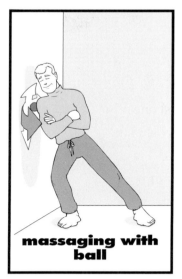

massaging with
ball

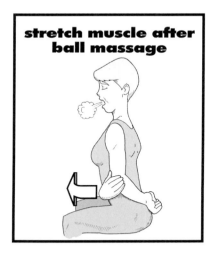

stretch muscle after
ball massage

body. Symptoms may include fever, increased pain, nausea, and vomiting.

Then turn to the sections of the book that describe how to stretch these muscles. Learn and perform these stretches as discussed and diagrammed. It will usually be easier to stretch **after** using the ball to stimulate blood flow and to push on trigger points. In this fashion, the myofascial component of a pain pattern can often be reduced and controlled most of the time.

BACKGROUND

Most of the time we can tell where we feel the pain in our body. We can tell that our shoulder hurts, head throbs, or lower back aches. We can differentiate among a knife-like pain by the shoulder blade, tingling in the thigh, and numbness in the hand. It is more difficult, however, to find the source of this pain. Before we accept that we are doomed by the pain of arthritis, the stiffness of old age, or the aches from an old sports injury, it is to our great advantage to try to understand the concepts of myofascial pain. With this knowledge it is possible to gain control of pain symptoms that have remained a mystery to both patients and medical care givers.

We can tell the location of pain symptoms and discomfort by simply knowing where we hurt. This is generally straightforward. Then we assume that the pain is caused by a problem or abnormality in the location or part of the body where the pain is located—and there might actually even be something wrong with your body in this area. A doctor may have diagnosed arthritis because of x-ray evidence of degenerative change. An MRI scan may have demonstrated disc problems. The television advertisement may have explained that your headache is coming from your sinuses. Believing these explanations and theories for the cause of your pain leads you to purchase the same remedies over and over again. We learn to live with these conditions believing we are at the mercy of an aging and injured body. Believing these theories as an explanation for pain symptoms may lead to surgery and other procedures that seldom eliminate the symptoms.

As you use this book, it is important to understand that *your pain does not always originate from the area where you feel the symptoms*. Not only that, but the source of this pain may be elusive and is generally not intuitive. *The pain may not only come from somewhere that does not hurt as much, it may even come from many places at once.*

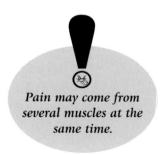

Pain may come from several muscles at the same time.

Myofascial pain does not only originate in the painful area. The pain may come from trigger points located in several muscles that act together as a functional unit to move a particular part of the body. It may also come from more distant muscles. These trigger points are like musical instruments in an orchestra that perform together to produce your pain pattern. With a longer duration of pain symptoms, more muscles are likely to become involved in generating a particular pain pattern (see "satellite trigger points" page 19). Usually, there is only a short period of time (minutes to hours) after injury when the pain might be caused by only one muscle or trigger point.

HEAD and NECK PAIN

Head and neck pain is generated by trigger points in the many muscles in the face, jaw, head, and neck. In addition, muscles in the upper shoulders and upper back can be the foundation or "cornerstone" for headache pain and neck stiffness. The most important outer area muscle to treat for head and neck pain is the infraspinatus muscle that is located on the shoulder blade (see pages 43 and 53). Occasionally, a calf muscle will refer pain to the face and jaw on the same side of the body (see page 39).

Sternocleidomastoid

The **sternocleidomastoid** muscle is located in the front and side of the neck, attaching to the sternum and clavicle in front, and to the mastoid process at the back side of the skull (see diagram **m-1**). It acts to turn and tilt the head, and lifts the head when doing a sit-up. Trigger points in this muscle usually refer pain to the cheek, ear, forehead, and the back of the head (see diagram **m-2**). They can also refer pain to the opposite side of the forehead. In addition, trigger points in this muscle can cause ringing in the ears (tinnitus) and difficulties with sense of balance. They can even cause vertigo. Trigger points in this muscle are usually a significant contributing cause of migraine headache. This muscle is easily injured during an automobile accident when a vehicle is struck from behind. Chewing gum and talking on the telephone will aggravate trigger points in this muscle.

Scalene

The **scalene** muscles are located along the side of the neck (see diagram **m-3**). They attach to the sides of the upper cervical vertebrae and to the first

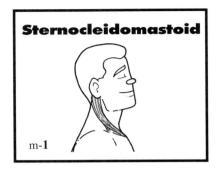

Sternocleidomastoid

m-1

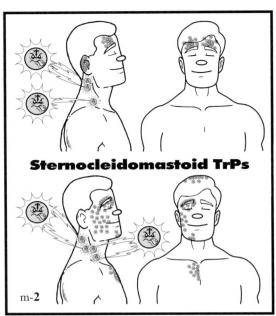

Sternocleidomastoid TrPs

m-2

and second ribs. Their action is to tilt the head sideways. Trigger points in this muscle refer pain, numbness, and tingling up into the face and head and down into the arm and hand (see diagram **m-4**). They can also refer pain

Scalene

m-3

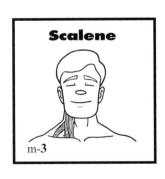

Scalene TrPs

m-4

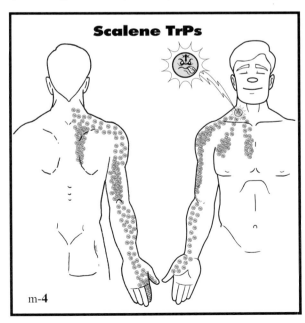

into the ear and may cause tinnitus. These muscles are especially injured by rapid head motion to the side and by sustained posture (staying in one position too long). Using the telephone and sleeping in an awkward position will often aggravate trigger points in these muscles.

Posterior Cervical and Suboccipital

Posterior cervical and suboccipital muscles are located in the back of the neck. They attach to the base of the skull and to the back of the cervical and upper thoracic vertebrae (see diagram **m-5**). Their action is to tilt the head backwards and keep it from falling forwards. Trigger points in these muscles typically cause headache pain that radiates up the back of the head,

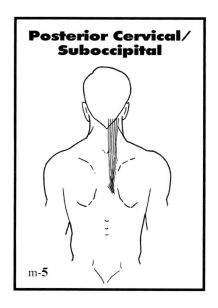

Posterior Cervical/ Suboccipital

m-**5**

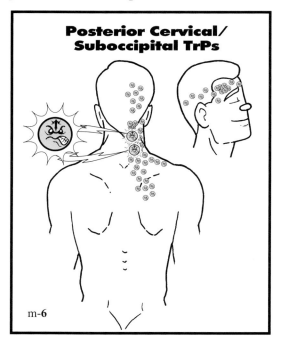

Posterior Cervical/ Suboccipital TrPs

m-**6**

around the side of the head, and into the forehead. They may also send pain down into the upper back (see diagram **m-6**). Pushing firmly on these muscles during a headache will be painful at first, and then the headache may be relieved. Physical activities that require a forward leaning head posture will often aggravate trigger points in these muscles.

Masseter and Temporalis

The **masseter** (see diagram **m-7**) and **temporalis** (see diagram **m-8**) muscles attach to the side of the face and head, and to the jaw bone. They are the primary muscles involved with biting and chewing. Trigger points in the masseter and temporalis muscles cause much of the pain of TMJ (now TMD) related disorders. They typically refer pain to the teeth, ear, side of the face, and jaw joint (see diagrams **m-9** and **m-10**). Trigger points in these muscles are *greatly aggravated by chewing gum*. They also tighten if there are active trigger points in the sternocleidomastoid and scalene muscles.

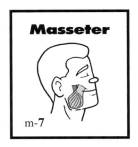

Masseter

m-7

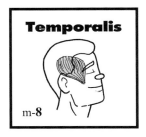

Temporalis

m-8

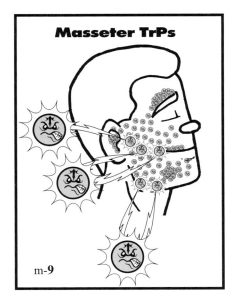

Masseter TrPs

m-9

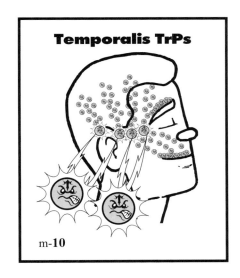

Temporalis TrPs

m-10

Trapezius

The **trapezius** muscle is large and covers the upper back, upper shoulder, and the back of the neck (see diagram **m-11**). Its actions include stabilizing and moving the head, neck, and upper shoulders. Trapezius muscle trigger points cause pain in the head, neck, and upper shoulders (see diagram **m-12** and **m-13**). Occasionally trigger points in these muscles will also refer pain into the upper arm. If any part of the muscle is tight and causing pain, the entire muscle may need to be treated in order to alleviate the pain pattern. Trigger points in this muscle are aggravated by tilting the head backwards, forward leaning posture, and working with the arms held above chest height.

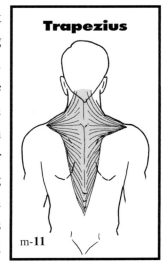

Trapezius

m-11

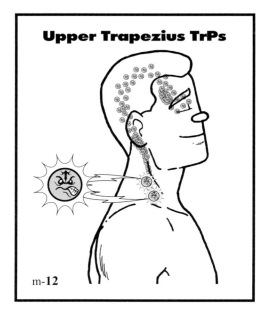

Upper Trapezius TrPs

m-12

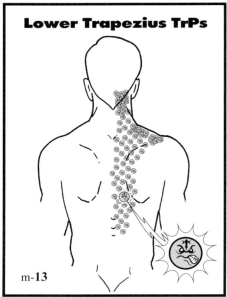

Lower Trapezius TrPs

m-13

Levator Scapulae

The **levator scapulae** muscle attaches to the upper inside corner of the shoulder blade and inserts on the side of the upper four cervical vertebrae (see diagram **m-14**). This muscle elevates the shoulder blade. It also assists with neck rotation. Trigger points in this muscle generate a pain pattern that

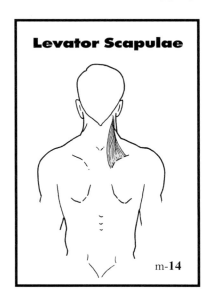

Levator Scapulae

m-14

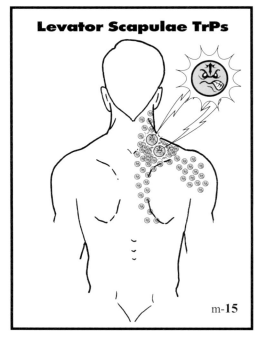

Levator Scapulae TrPs

m-15

is felt in the corner between the neck and upper shoulder and down along the inside border of the shoulder blade (see diagram **m-15**). This muscle is usually involved in symptoms that are described as a "stiff neck." Trigger points in this muscle are aggravated by carrying objects, wearing a back pack or a purse, awkward neck postures, and working with the arms held above chest height.

Soleus

The **soleus** muscle attaches to the back of the calf and to the back of the heel (see diagram **m-16**). It acts to push the foot down (gas pedal).

Trigger points in the soleus muscle can refer pain to the jaw and side of the face (see diagram **m-17**). They will be aggravated by walking and running. If face and jaw pain is unresponsive to treatment focused on the head, jaw, and neck, this source of pain should be considered. Treatment may involve shoe inserts and body work on the feet and calves.

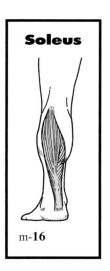

Soleus

m-**16**

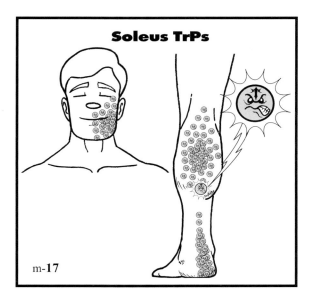

Soleus TrPs

m-**17**

SHOULDER PAIN

Shoulder pain is generated by trigger points in the many muscles that work together to move the shoulder. These primarily include the trapezius, deltoid, pectoralis, biceps, triceps, latissimus, and the muscles of the rotator cuff. The rotator cuff muscles include the supraspinatus, infraspinatus, subscapularis, and teres minor. They are called rotator cuff muscles because their main function is to rotate the upper arm. A rotator cuff tear can perpetuate myofascial trigger points in any of these muscles. Whether an MRI scan is positive or negative for a tear in the rotator cuff tendon, a major part of the shoulder pain is likely to be generated by myofascial trigger points in several of these muscles. Techniques described in this book can help treat them. If the medical diagnosis is "frozen shoulder" syndrome, work should be concentrated on infraspinatus, upper latissimus, and supraspinatus musculature.

Trapezius

The **trapezius** muscle is large and covers the upper back, upper shoulder, and the back of the neck (see diagram **m-18**). Its actions include stabilizing and moving the head, neck, and upper shoulders. Trapezius muscle trigger points cause pain in the head, neck, and upper shoulders (see diagram **m-19**). Occasionally trigger points in these muscles will also refer pain into the upper arm. If any part of the muscle is tight and causing pain, the entire muscle may need to be treated in order to alleviate the pain pattern. Trigger points in this muscle are aggravated by tilting the head backwards, forward leaning posture, and working with the arms held above chest height.

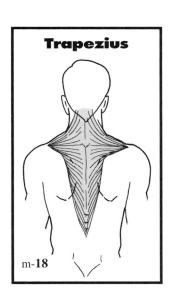

Trapezius

m-18

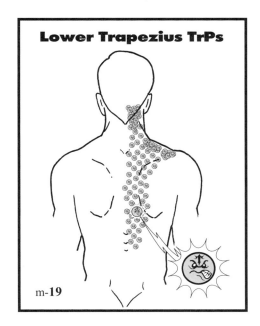

Lower Trapezius TrPs

m-19

Deltoid

The **deltoid** muscle covers the top, side, front, and back of the shoulder joint (see diagram **m-20**). There are three parts to this muscle, and they contract to move the arm away from the body in any direction including front, side, and behind. Trigger points in this muscle cause pain that radiates into the shoulder joint and the upper arm (see diagrams **m-21** and **m-22**). They

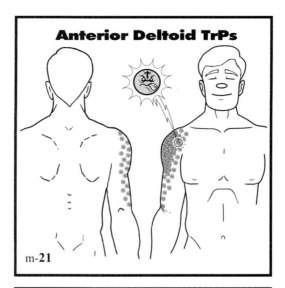

Anterior Deltoid TrPs

m-21

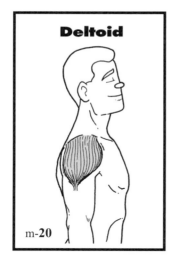

Deltoid

m-20

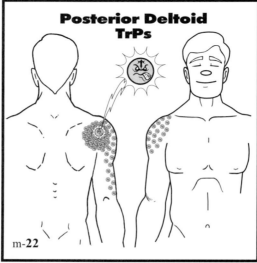

Posterior Deltoid TrPs

m-22

are aggravated by moving the arm out and up in any direction. These trigger points may also be activated by trauma and bruising, and also by injection of medication. The front and back parts of the muscle can be adequately stretched, but the middle part may respond best to using the ball and injection techniques.

Supraspinatus

The **supraspinatus** muscle fits in a groove across the upper part of the shoulder blade (see diagram **m-23**). It acts primarily to move the arm out sideways from the body. Trigger points in this muscle refer pain into the upper shoulder, arm, and neck (see diagram **m-24**). They will contribute to "stiff neck" symptoms. Moving the arm out to the side and upwards and working with the arms above chest height can aggravate these trigger points.

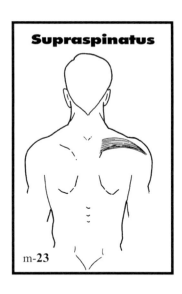

Supraspinatus

m-23

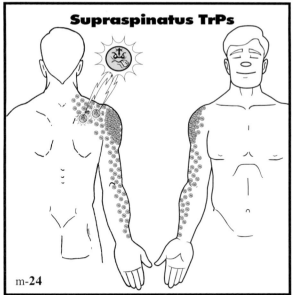

Supraspinatus TrPs

m-24

Infraspinatus

The **infraspinatus** muscle is located over the lower two thirds of the shoulder blade and inserts on the back of the upper arm (see diagram **m-25**).

Contraction of this muscle stabilizes the shoulder joint and rotates the upper arm outward and to the side. Trigger points in this muscle cause pain in the upper back and refer pain into the arm, forearm, hand, outer shoulder, front of the shoulder, upper shoulder, and neck (see diagram **m-26**). They can also refer pain to the other side of the body. In addition, they may cause numbness and tingling in the forearm, ring, and small fingers. Trigger points

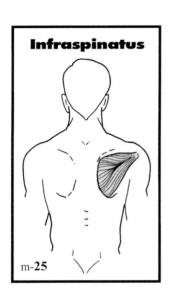

Infraspinatus

m-25

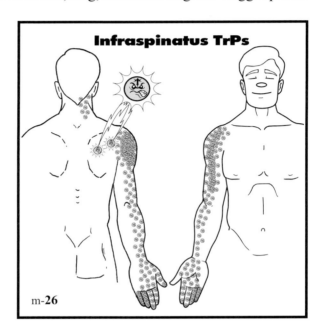

Infraspinatus TrPs

m-26

in this muscle are a major part of "frozen shoulder" syndrome, and are indeed the cornerstone for neck stiffness, neck pain, headache, and migraine. Latent trigger points will subtly decrease shoulder motion in internal rotation. When this muscle's flexibility is normal, it should be possible to place the fingers of the right hand behind the back and up to the level of the bottom of the left shoulder blade. Lastly, this muscle is relatively weak for the work it is often asked to perform. Activities such as pushing open a car door from inside the car, holding open a self-closing store door, or separating tightly packed clothing that is hanging in a closet all aggravate trigger points in this muscle.

Subscapularis

The **subscapularis** muscle lines the underside of the shoulder blade over the rib cage, and attaches to the upper arm (see diagram **m-27**). It internally rotates and pulls the arm down. It also helps hold the shoulder blade to the chest. It is used in holding and carrying with two arms, pulling objects from the side, shivering when cold, and hugging. Trigger points in this muscle refer deep pain into the upper back, chest, shoulder, forearm, and wrist (see diagram **m-28**). Trigger points in this muscle also are a major factor in "frozen shoulder." This is aggravated by throwing, and usually gets very sore after the first baseball or football throws of the season.

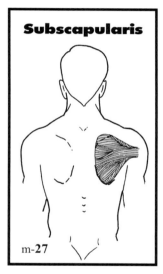

Subscapularis

m-27

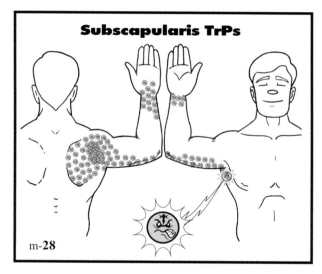

Subscapularis TrPs

m-28

Teres Minor

The **teres minor** muscle is located in the side of the mid to upper back between the shoulder blade and the back of the upper arm (see diagram **m-29**). Contraction of this muscle rotates the arm outward and stabilizes the shoulder joint. Trigger points in this muscle cause pain in the back of the shoulder and into the upper outer arm (see diagram **m-30**). Pushing open a car door from inside the car, holding open a self-closing store door, and separating

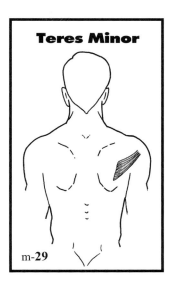

Teres Minor

m-29

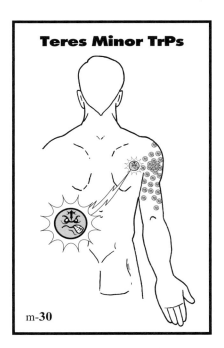

Teres Minor TrPs

m-30

tightly packed clothing that is hanging in a closet all aggravate trigger points in this muscle.

Teres Major

The **teres major** muscle is located in the side of the back between the upper arm and the shoulder blade (see diagram **m-31**). It attaches to the shoulder blade and the upper arm. Contraction of this muscle rotates the arm inward, pulls the arm in towards the body, and helps pull the arm backward when it is in front of the body. Trigger points in this muscle cause pain in the back of the shoulder and into the back of the arm and forearm (see diagram **m-32**). Pain symptoms can be caused by reaching forward and up. These trigger points are aggravated by tensing while driving and by driving an automobile that is difficult to steer.

45

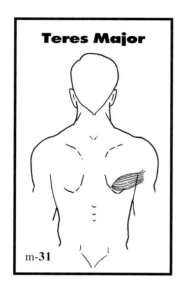

Teres Major

m-31

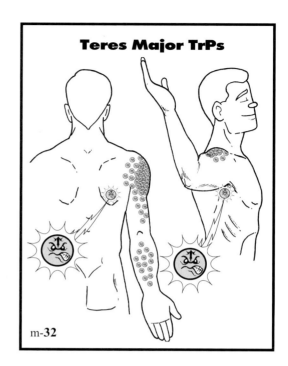

Teres Major TrPs

m-32

Upper Latissimus

The **upper latissimus** muscle is located along the back and side of the body (see diagram **m-33**). It goes from the spinous processes of the lower six thoracic vertebrae and all of the lumbar vertebrae and attaches to the upper arm above and the pelvic bones below. The spinous processes are the parts of each vertebrae that can be felt under the skin in the middle all down the back. Contraction of this muscle pulls the arm downward, stabilizes the shoulder blade, and assists in rotating the arm inward and pulling the arms backward. Trigger points in this muscle refer pain into the arm, around the shoulder blade to the back of the shoulder, around the chest into the inner arm, and down into the hand, and fingers (see diagram **m-34**). These trigger points can cause the sharp chest pain that is often called pleurisy. These trigger points are aggravated by doing chin-ups, walking with crutches, carrying objects under your arm, and shivering.

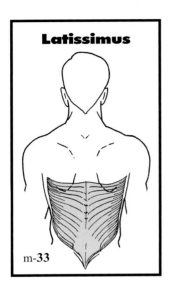

Latissimus

m-**33**

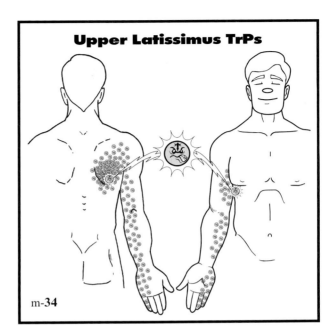

Upper Latissimus TrPs

m-**34**

Pectoralis

The **pectoralis** muscle is located over the front of the chest and upper arm (see diagram **m-35**). It attaches the ribs, breast , and collar bones to the upper arm. Contraction of this muscle brings the shoulder blade forward, rotates the arm inward, and brings the arm across the chest. It is used to push forward, draw inward, stabilize the shoulder, and hug. Trigger points in this muscle cause pain in the front of the chest, upper arm, elbow, hand, and fingers (see diagram **m-36** and **m-37**). These trigger points may contribute to "carpal tunnel" symptoms. They may also be part of irregular heart beat and chest

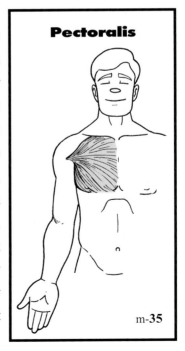

Pectoralis

m-**35**

map

pain symptoms. Pain symptoms may be aggravated by pushing away from the body and raking,

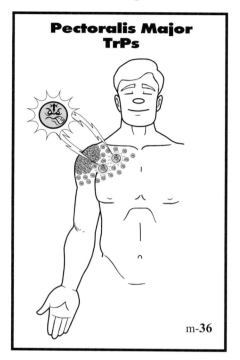

Pectoralis Major TrPs

m-36

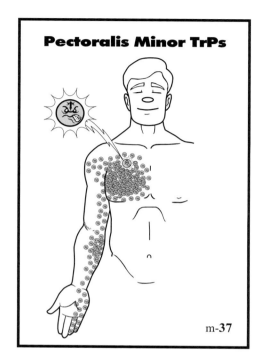

Pectoralis Minor TrPs

m-37

Biceps

The **biceps** muscle is located along the front of the upper arm (see diagram **m-38**). It attaches the front of the shoulder blade to the front of the forearm near the elbow. Contraction of this muscle bends the elbow and rotates the wrist outwards. Trigger points in this muscle cause pain, numbness and tingling in the front of the arm, and refer pain from the front of the shoulder to the front of the elbow. (see diagram **m-39**). Carpal tunnel syndrome is often caused initially by tightness and trigger points in these muscles. These trigger points will

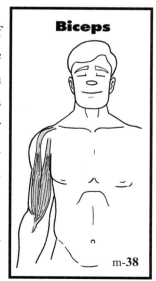

Biceps

m-38

be aggravated by holding objects, carrying, climbing (a rope or ladder), and using a screw driver. This is the major muscle that is used when the right hand tightens a screw, or the left hand loosens a screw.

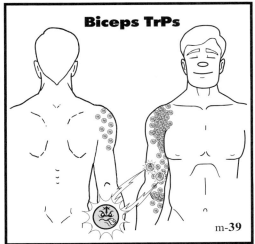

Biceps TrPs

m-39

Triceps

The **triceps** muscle is located along the back of the upper arm (see diagram **m-40**). It attaches the upper arm and shoulder blade to the forearm at the back of the elbow. Contraction of this muscle primarily straightens the elbow. Trigger points in this muscle cause pain in the upper posterior arm,

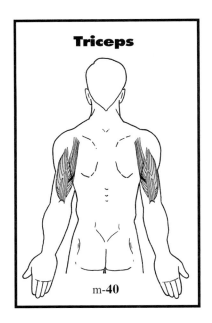

Triceps

m-40

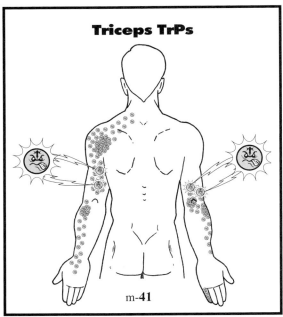

Triceps TrPs

m-41

49

and refer pain to the shoulder joint, upper shoulder, posterior elbow, forearm, and fourth and fifth fingers (see diagram **m-41**). They will be aggravated by punching, pushing objects, and doing push-ups.

ARM PAIN

Arm pain is generated by trigger points in the many muscles that work together to move the shoulder, elbow, wrist, and fingers. These primarily include the infraspinatus, subscapularis, upper latissimus, teres, brachialis, biceps, triceps, and forearm muscles. Trigger points in these muscles can cause numbness and tingling from the shoulder to the fingers, a deep ache, sharp and severe pain, cramping, and weakness. They can also make the arm feel heavy. Some of these muscles also contribute to shoulder pain and are discussed in both sections.

Biceps

The **biceps** muscle is located along the front of the upper arm (see diagram **m-42**). It attaches the front of the shoulder blade to the front of the forearm near the elbow. Contraction of this muscle bends the elbow and rotates the wrist outwards. Trigger points in this muscle cause pain, numbness and tingling in the front of the arm, and refer pain from the front of the shoulder to the front of the elbow. (see diagram **m-43**). Carpal tunnel syndrome is often caused initially by tightness and trigger points in these muscles. These trigger points will be aggravated by

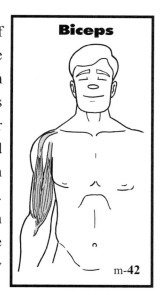

Biceps

m-42

holding objects, carrying, climbing (a rope or ladder), and using a screw driver. This is the major muscle that is used when the right hand tightens a screw, or the left hand loosens a screw.

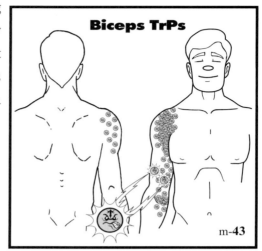

m-43

Triceps

The **triceps** muscle is located along the back of the upper arm (see diagram **m-44**). It attaches the upper arm and shoulder blade to the forearm at the back of the elbow. Contraction of this muscle primarily straightens the elbow. Trigger points in this muscle cause pain in the upper posterior arm,

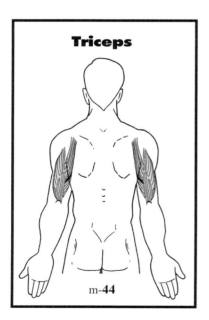

m-44

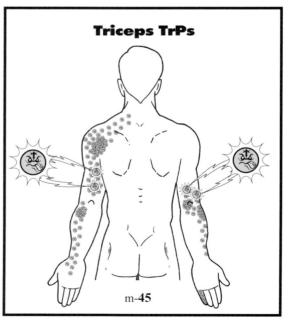

m-45

and refer pain to the shoulder joint, upper shoulder, posterior elbow, forearm, and fourth and fifth fingers (see diagram **m-45**). They will be aggravated by punching, pushing objects, and doing push-ups.

Brachialis

The **brachialis** muscle is located along the front of the arm and goes from the upper arm to the radius bone in the forearm (see diagram **m-46**). Contraction of this muscle primarily bends the elbow. Trigger points in this muscle refer pain from the front of the shoulder, along the front of the arm into the elbow, and into the area of the thumb joint at the wrist and first thumb knuckle (see diagram **m-47**). This muscle remains contracted in order to support the hand and fingers during physical activity such as typing or working on objects at waist level. It also contracts to do chin-ups. Trigger points in this muscle will be aggravated by holding and carrying things with the elbow bent and desk work such as typing (if upper extremities are not well supported).

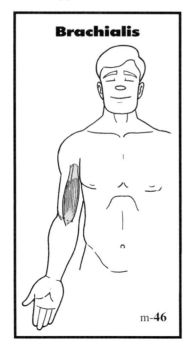

Brachialis

m-46

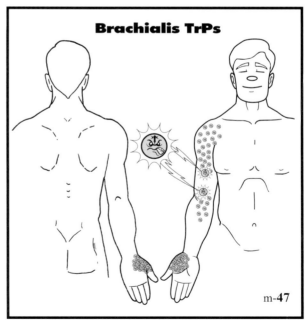

Brachialis TrPs

m-47

Infraspinatus

The **infraspinatus** muscle is located over the lower two thirds of the shoulder blade and inserts on the back of the upper arm (see diagram **m-48**). Contraction of this muscle stabilizes the shoulder joint and rotates the upper arm outward and to the side. Trigger points in this muscle cause pain in the upper back and refer pain into the arm, forearm, hand, outer shoulder, front of the shoulder, upper shoulder, and neck (see diagram **m-49**). They can also refer pain to the other side of the body. In addition, they may cause numbness and tingling in the forearm, ring and small fingers. Trigger points in this muscle are a major part of "frozen shoulder"

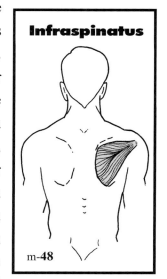

Infraspinatus

m-**48**

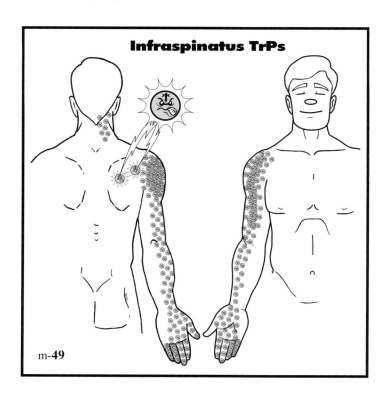

Infraspinatus TrPs

m-**49**

syndrome, and are indeed the cornerstone for neck stiffness, neck pain, headache, and migraine. Latent trigger points will subtly decrease shoulder motion in internal rotation. When this muscle's flexibility is normal, it should be possible to place the fingers of the right hand behind the back and up to the level of the bottom of the left shoulder blade. Lastly, this muscle is relatively weak for the work it is often asked to perform. Activities such as pushing open a car door from inside the car, holding open a self-closing store door, or separating tightly packed clothing that is hanging in a closet all aggravate trigger points in this muscle.

Teres minor

The **teres minor** muscle is located in the side of the mid to upper back between the shoulder blade and the back of the upper arm (see diagram **m-50**).

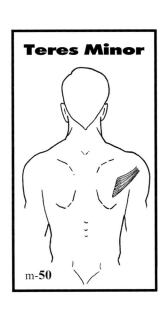

Teres Minor

m-**50**

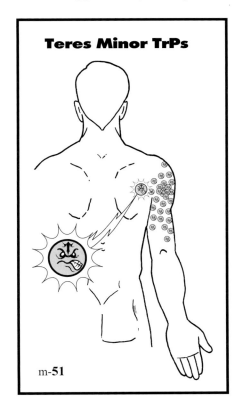

Teres Minor TrPs

m-**51**

Contraction of this muscle rotates the arm outward and stabilizes the shoulder joint. Trigger points in this muscle cause pain in the back of the shoulder and into the upper outer arm (see diagram **m-51**). Activities such as pushing open a car door from inside the car, holding open a self-closing store door, or separating tightly packed clothing that is hanging in a closet all aggravate trigger points in this muscle.

Upper Latissimus

The **upper latissimus** muscle is located along the back and side of the body (see diagram **m-52**). It goes from the spinous processes of the lower six thoracic vertebrae and all of the lumbar vertebrae and attaches to the upper arm above and the pelvic bones below. The spinous process is the part of each vertebrae that can be felt under the skin, in the middle, all down the back. Contraction of this muscle pulls the arm downward, stabilizes the shoulder blade, and assists in rotating the arm inward and pulling the arms backward. Trigger points in this muscle refer pain into the arm, around the

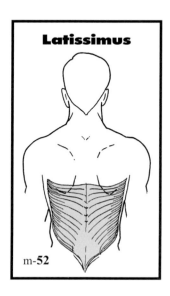

Latissimus

m-**52**

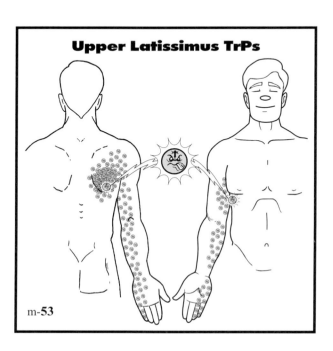

Upper Latissimus TrPs

m-**53**

shoulder blade to the back of the shoulder, around the chest into the inner arm, and down into the hand and fingers (see diagram **m-53**). These trigger points can cause the sharp chest pain that is often called pleurisy. These trigger points are aggravated by doing chin-ups, walking with crutches, carrying objects under your arm, and shivering.

Subscapularis

The **subscapularis** muscle lines the underside of the shoulder blade over the rib cage, and attaches to the upper arm (see diagram **m-54**). It internally rotates and pulls the arm down. It also helps hold the shoulder blade to the chest. Trigger points in this muscle refer deep pain into the upper back, chest,

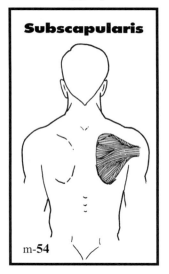

Subscapularis

m-54

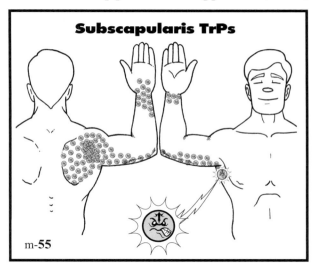

Subscapularis TrPs

m-55

shoulder, forearm, and wrist (see diagram **m-55**). They are also a major factor in "frozen shoulder." The pain from these trigger points is aggravated by holding and carrying objects with two arms, pulling objects from the side, shivering when cold, hugging, and throwing. The first baseball or football throws of the season can cause considerable soreness in this muscle.

ELBOW PAIN/WRIST PAIN

Elbow and wrist pain are generated by trigger points in the many muscles that work together to move the elbow, shoulder, wrist, and fingers. These primarily include the biceps, triceps, wrist extensors, wrist flexors, supinator, and pronator teres. Other muscles that refer pain to this area include infraspinatus, upper latissimus, and scalene muscles discussed above. "Tennis elbow" pain is typically generated by wrist extensors and supinator muscles. "Golfer's elbow" is typically generated by wrist flexors. Both of these conditions often result from trigger points in the tendon of origin (at the bony attachment to the elbow), and in the muscle belly. Your efforts should focus on the techniques for treating the muscle belly.

Wrist Extensors (Dorsiflexors)

These muscles include the **brachioradialis**, **extensor carpi radialis brevis**, **extensor carpi radialis longus**, and **extensor carpi ulnaris** (see diagram **m-56**). They attach to the outside areas of the bones of the arm and forearm at the elbow joint, and also to the top side of the end of the forearm, or wrist and hand bones. The primary action of these muscles is to bend the wrist backwards. Trigger points in these muscles refer pain to the back of the elbow, top of the wrist, thumb side of the forearm, and between the thumb

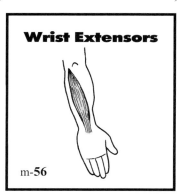

Wrist Extensors

m-56

and index fingers (see diagram **m-57**). They are usually involved in causing the pain of tennis elbow. These trigger points can be aggravated by other forearm and finger activities such as typing, craft work, and assembly.

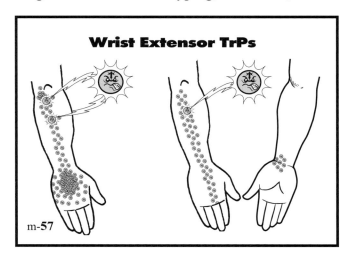

m-57

Wrist Flexors (Palmar Flexors)

These muscles include the **palmaris longus**, **flexor carpi radialis**, and **flexor carpi ulnaris** (see diagram **m-58** and **m-60**). They attach to the inside

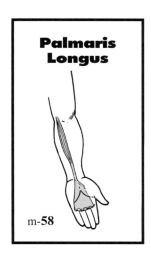

m-58

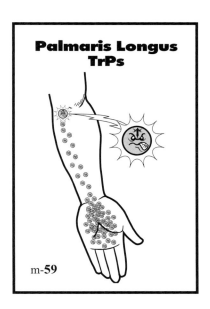

m-59

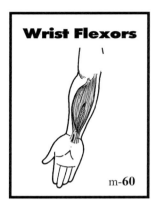

Wrist Flexors

m-60

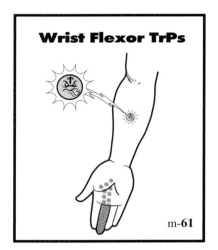

Wrist Flexor TrPs

m-61

areas of the bones of the arm and forearm at the elbow joint, and also to the palm side of the end of the forearm, wrist, and hand bones. The action of these muscles is to bend the wrist toward the palm side of the hand. Trigger points in these muscles refer pain to the forearm, wrist, palm, and the inside of the elbow (see diagram **m-59** and **m-61**). They are often involved in causing the pain of "golfer's elbow." These trigger points can be aggravated by other forearm and finger activities such as typing, craft work, and assembly.

Supinator

The **supinator** muscle attaches to the outside of the elbow at the end of the upper arm and to the radius and ulna bones of the forearm (see diagram **m-62**). Its primary action is to twist the wrist to the outside, clockwise for the right hand and counterclockwise for the left hand. Trigger points in this muscle refer pain to the outside of the elbow and into the hand between the wrist, thumb, and index fingers (see diagram **m-63**). This muscle is usually involved in causing the pain of tennis elbow. These trigger points will also be aggravated by craft work, assembly, and turning a screw driver.

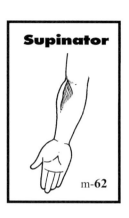

Supinator

m-62

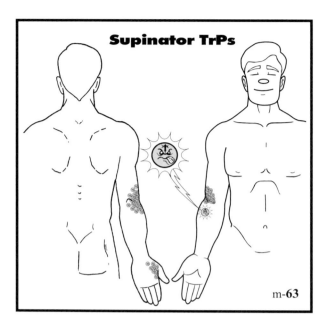

Supinator TrPs

m-63

Pronator Teres

The **pronator teres** muscle starts at the inside of the elbow at the end of the upper arm and attaches to the outside of the radius bone in the forearm (see diagram **m-64**). This muscle rotates and turns the hand downward and

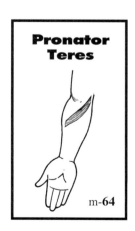

Pronator Teres

m-64

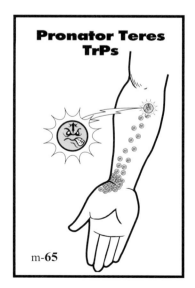

Pronator Teres TrPs

m-65

inward. It turns the right hand counterclockwise and the left-hand clockwise. Trigger points in this muscle refer pain into the palm side of the forearm and over towards the thumb side of the wrist (see diagram **m-65**). This muscle is usually involved in causing the pain of "golfer's elbow." These trigger points will also be aggravated by craft work, assembly, and turning a screw driver.

FOREARM PAIN

Forearm pain is generated by trigger points in the many muscles that work together to move the neck, shoulder, elbow, wrist, and fingers. The muscles that move the neck, shoulder, and elbow primarily include the scalene, infraspinatus, upper latissimus, biceps, and triceps discussed previously. The other major muscles that cause forearm pain rotate the forearm and move the wrist and fingers. On the top side of the forearm these include the wrist extensors as listed and described previously. On the palm side of the forearm are the wrist flexors, as listed and described previously, and the palmaris longus muscle. The wrist flexors also contribute to carpal tunnel syndrome (see page 174).

Palmaris Longus

The **palmaris longus** starts at the inside of the elbow and attaches to the deep and thick protective fascia of the palm and the transverse carpal ligament that covers the palm side of the wrist (see diagram **m-66**). These structures keep the skin of the palm tight and form the palm side of the carpal tunnel. This muscle cups the palm and assists in bending the wrist. Trigger points in this muscle refer pain along the palm side of the forearm and into the center of the palm (see diagram **m-67**). The pain sensation may feel like a painful prickle close to the skin. These trigger points can be aggravated by

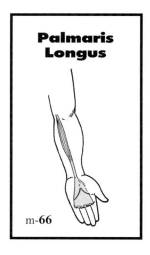

Palmaris Longus

m-66

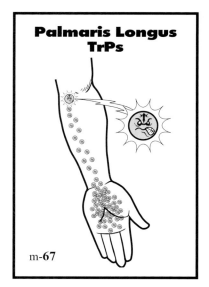

Palmaris Longus TrPs

m-67

activities that require hand grip, wrist and hand motion, and carrying with the fingers.

HAND and FINGER PAIN

Hand pain and finger pain, including numbness and tingling, can be generated by trigger points in the muscles of the shoulder girdle and arm as described previously. More intense pain in the hand and fingers is usually generated by the muscles in the forearm and hand that make the fingers move.

Forearm muscles on the palm side that move the fingers include flexor digitorum superficialis, flexor digitorum profundus, and flexor pollicis longus. These muscles refer pain to the thumb and fingers. Sometimes this is described as a lightning pain that may feel as if it is going *beyond* the tips of the fingers. Trigger points in these muscles also contribute to the conditions called trigger finger and Dupuytren's contracture. Though these conditions are not discussed in this book, following the stretching and massage instructions here is likely to be helpful.

First Web Space

The **first web space** is the area of the hand between the bones of the thumb and the bones of the index finger (see diagram **m-68**). These bones are called the first and second metacarpals. The muscles include the adductor pollicis and opponens pollicis. Their primary action is to move the thumb so the hand can hold objects. Trigger points in these muscles generate pain in the area of the thumb and the fifth finger side of the hand (see diagram **m-71**) and are often involved in writer's cramp. They will be aggravated by writing, working with scissors, and sustained gripping.

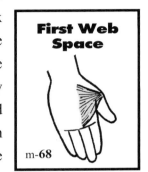

First Web Space

m-68

Adductor Pollicis

The **adductor pollicis** starts at the base of the thumb and attaches to the second and third metacarpal bones and the capitate bone of the wrist (see diagram **m-69**). Contraction of this muscle brings the thumb toward the index finger. It also assists in bending the thumb. Trigger points in this muscle generate pain in the area of the thumb and the fifth finger side of the hand (see diagram **m-71**). They will be especially aggravated by gripping small objects.

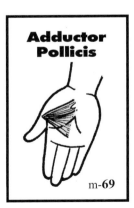

Adductor Pollicis

m-69

Opponens Pollicis

The **opponens pollicis** muscle starts at the trapezoid bone of the wrist

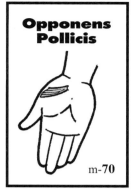

Opponens Pollicis

m-70

and the palmar wrist ligament, and attaches to the first metacarpal thumb bone in the palm (see diagram **m-70**). This muscle rotates the thumb into a position where the hand can pinch and grasp an object. Trigger points in this muscle refer pain to the thumb, wrist, and fifth finger side of the hand (see diagram **m-71**). They will be aggravated by writing, holding, and gripping.

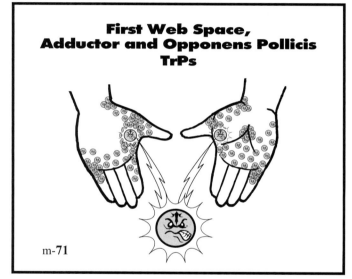

First Web Space, Adductor and Opponens Pollicis TrPs

m-71

Lumbricals (Intrinsic Muscles)

The **lumbrical** and **intrinsic** muscles of the hand start at the metacarpal bones and attach to the finger bones or the finger extensor tendons (see diagram **m-72**). Contraction of these muscles separates the fingers, bends the knuckles, and straightens the fingers. Trigger points in these muscles generate pain in the areas of the palm, top of the hand, and into the fingers and finger joints (see diagram **m-73**). They also cause stiffness and dexterity problems. Activities that involve repetitive finger motion and gripping will tend to aggravate these trigger points.

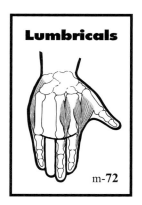

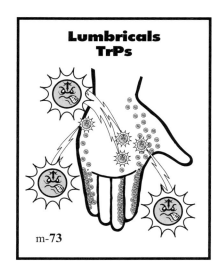

UPPER BACK PAIN

Upper back pain is generated by trigger points in the muscles that hold and stabilize the shoulder blade, muscles that move the shoulder, muscles that move the spine, and muscles that move the ribs. Some of these muscles also generate referral pain patterns that are felt in the shoulder, neck, arm, forearm, or hand. These muscles include the levator scapulae, supraspinatus, infraspinatus, latissimus dorsi, rhomboid, serratus posterior superior, upper paraspinal, middle and lower trapezius and intercostal muscles. The most important trigger points, and the cornerstone for upper back pain are in the infraspinatus muscle. Even though they may be latent and not tender, be sure to include using the ball and stretch techniques on these muscles whenever you are treating pain in the upper back.

Levator Scapulae

The **levator scapulae muscle** attaches to the upper inside corner of the shoulder blade, and inserts on the side of the upper four cervical vertebrae (see diagram **m-74**). This muscle elevates the shoulder blade, and it also assists with neck rotation. Trigger points in this muscle refer pain to the corner between the neck and upper shoulder and down along the inside border of the shoulder blade (see diagram **m-75**). This muscle is usually involved in symptoms that are described as a "stiff neck." These trigger points will be aggravated by reaching above shoulder height, carrying objects with the arms, keyboard work without chair arm support, wearing a back pack, and wearing a purse on the shoulder.

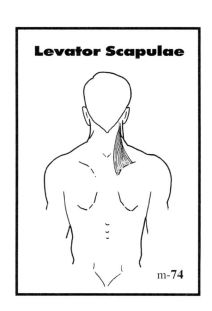

m-74

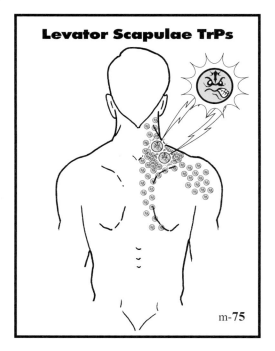

m-75

Supraspinatus

The **supraspinatus** muscle fits in a groove across the upper part of the shoulder blade (see diagram **m-76**). It acts primarily to move the arm out sideways from the body. Trigger points in this muscle refer pain into the upper shoulder, arm, and neck (see diagram **m-77**). They will contribute to "stiff neck" symptoms and pain across the upper shoulders. Moving the arm out to the side and upwards and working with the arms above chest height can aggravate these trigger points.

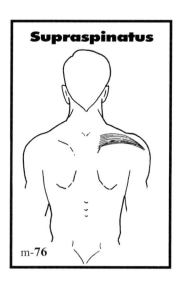

m-76

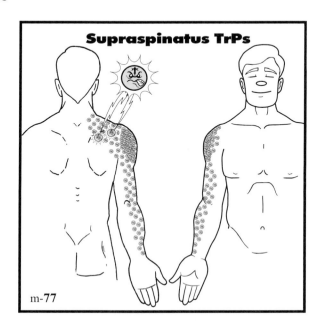

Supraspinatus TrPs

m-77

Infraspinatus

The **infraspinatus** muscle is located over the lower two thirds of the shoulder blade and inserts on the back of the upper arm (see diagram **m-78**). Contraction of this muscle stabilizes the shoulder joint and rotates the upper arm outward and to the side. Trigger points in this muscle cause pain in the upper back over the shoulder blade, between the shoulder blades, and over the spine. They also refer pain into the arm, forearm, hand, outer shoulder, front of the shoulder, upper shoulder, and neck (see diagram **m-79**). These trigger points can also refer pain to the other side of the body and upper back. Indeed, **trigger points in this muscle underlie and are the cornerstone foundation of many of the pain patterns that involve the upper back and**

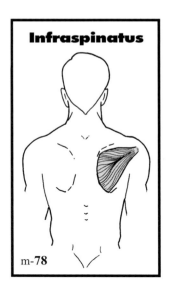

Infraspinatus

m-78

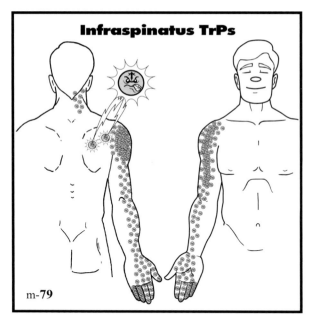

Infraspinatus TrPs

m-79

shoulder. When this muscle's flexibility is normal, it should be possible to place the fingers of the right hand behind the back and up to the level of the bottom of the left shoulder blade. Lastly, this muscle is relatively weak for the work it is often asked to perform. Activities such as pushing open a car door from inside the car, holding open a self-closing store door, or separating tightly packed clothing that is hanging in a closet all aggravate trigger points in this muscle.

Latissimus

The **latissimus** muscle is located along the back and sides of the body (see diagram **m-80**). It goes from the spinous processes of the lower six thoracic vertebrae and all of the lumbar vertebrae and attaches to the upper arm above and the pelvic bones below. The spinous process is the part of each vertebrae that can be felt under the skin, in the middle, all down the back. Contraction of this muscle pulls the arm downward, stabilizes the shoulder blade, and assists in rotating the arm inward and pulling the arms backward. Trigger points in this muscle refer pain into the arm, around the shoulder blade to the back of the shoulder, around the chest into the inner arm, around the chest and under the breast, and down into the hand and fingers (see diagram **m-81**). These trigger points can also cause the sharp chest pain that is often called pleurisy. These trigger points are aggravated by doing chin-ups, walking with crutches, carrying objects under your arm, and shivering.

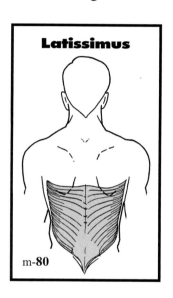

Latissimus

m-80

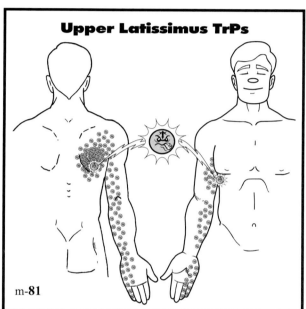

Upper Latissimus TrPs

m-81

Rhomboid

The **rhomboid** muscle starts at the inside border of the shoulder blade and attaches to the seventh cervical vertebrae and the first five thoracic vertebrae (see diagram **m-82**). These muscles are used to retract and stabilize the shoulder blade. Trigger points in this muscle refer pain along the inside border of the shoulder blade and into the back of the neck (see diagram **m-83**). They are aggravated by rowing and by holding the steering wheel tightly while driving. They will also be aggravated by tight pectoralis muscles which pull the shoulders forward and cause the rhomboids to work harder in an effort to balance the body by pulling the shoulders backward.

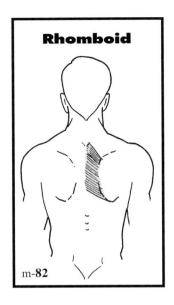

Rhomboid

m-**82**

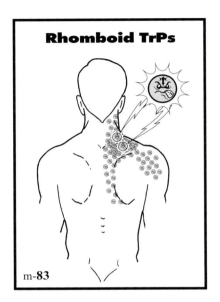

Rhomboid TrPs

m-**83**

Serratus Posterior Superior

The **serratus posterior superior** muscle starts at the inside border of the shoulder blade and attaches to the sixth and seventh cervical vertebrae and the first two thoracic vertebrae (see diagram **m-84**). It is located underneath the rhomboid muscles. This muscle is used to retract and stabilize the shoulder blade. Trigger points in this muscle generate pain over the shoulder blade, chest, and down into the arm and hand (see diagram **m-85**). They are aggravated by reaching to the side with the arms and by vigorous breathing and coughing.

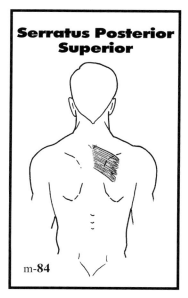

Serratus Posterior Superior

m-84

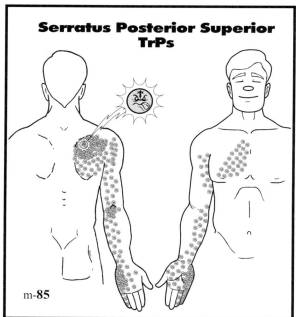

Serratus Posterior Superior TrPs

m-85

Paraspinal (Multifidus)

Upper (thoracic) paraspinal muscles attach to the vertebrae and the ribs. They are located right alongside the spine and assist with rotation of the spine (see diagram **m-86**). Trigger points in these muscles refer pain along the spine from the neck to the sacrum (see diagram **m-87**), and may even refer pain to the abdomen. They are aggravated by lifting, twisting, and repeated bending forward.

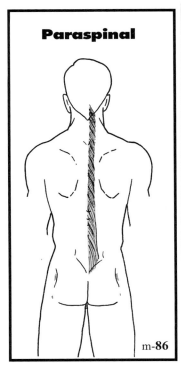

Paraspinal

m-86

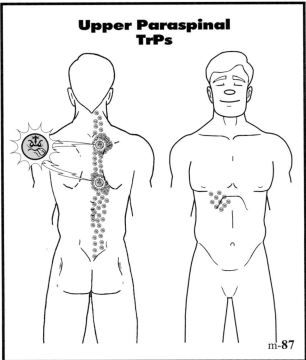

Upper Paraspinal TrPs

m-87

Middle and Lower Trapezius

The **middle and lower trapezius** muscle drapes across the upper shoulders, attaches to the shoulder blades, and inserts on the vertebrae from the top of the neck to the twelfth thoracic segment (see diagram **m-88**). These muscles are used to retract and lower the shoulder blade. Trigger points in this muscle generate pain from the middle back, to the shoulder blades, the back of the neck, and the base of the skull (see diagram **m-89**). They are aggravated by reaching forward, repeated bending, and working with the hands above chest height.

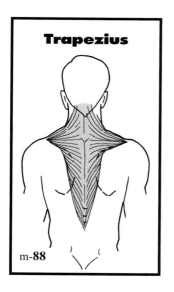

Trapezius

m-**88**

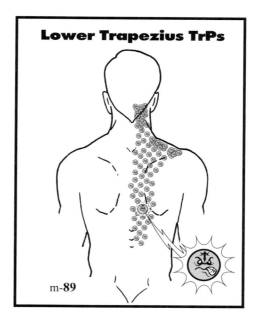

Lower Trapezius TrPs

m-**89**

Intercostal

Intercostal muscles attach to the ribs (see diagram **m-90**). These muscles serve to expand and contract the chest during breathing. Trigger points in these muscles cause pain in the back and around to the sides and front of the chest. Pain patterns are so varied that they are not illustrated here. The ball **should not** be used on these muscles because the ribs could be bruised or broken and the ball will not fit effectively between the ribs. The best stretches for these muscles are deep breathing exercises and latissimus stretches (see pages 152-155).

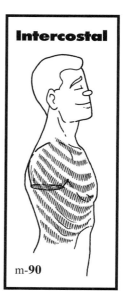

Intercostal

m-90

LOWER BACK PAIN

Lower back pain is generated by trigger points in the muscles that move the lower back and hip, and muscles that form the floor of the pelvis. Some of these muscles can also generate pain patterns that radiate up the back or down into the lower extremity. These include the quadratus lumborum, lower paraspinal, lower latissimus, rectus abdominus, iliopsoas, pelvic floor, gluteus maximus, gluteus medius, gluteus minimus and piriformis muscles. The most important trigger points and the cornerstone for lower back pain are in the gluteal muscles. Even though they may be latent and not tender, be sure to include using the ball and stretch techniques on these muscles whenever you are treating pain in the lower back. In addition, latent trigger points in hamstring muscles can perpetuate lower back pain. Treating these is also likely to be important (see page 93). Orthoses and shoe inserts may be especially helpful in treating lower back pain.

Quadratus Lumborum

The **quadratus lumborum** muscle attaches to the top of the pelvic bone, the lumbar vertebrae, and the 12th rib (see diagram **m-91**). This muscle functions to stabilize the lumbar spine, hike the hip, and bend the lower back sideways. Both sides of this muscle act together to bend the body backwards and to cough. The pain pattern from these trigger points can be felt in the mid back, lower back, buttocks, hip, and groin (see diagram **m-92**). Trigger points in this muscle can make coughing, sneezing, and going to the bathroom (defecation) extremely painful. These trigger points are often activated by bending and twisting at the same time. The human body is not designed to simultaneously bend, lift, and twist while carrying weight. This muscle is more likely to cause a pain flair after pushing a vacuum than after pushing a lawn mower.

74

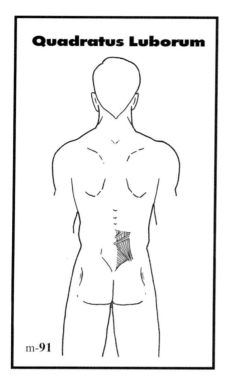

Quadratus Luborum

m-91

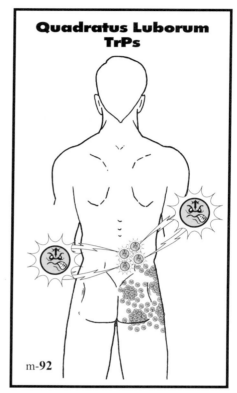

Quadratus Luborum TrPs

m-92

Paraspinal (Multifidus)

Lower (lumbar) **paraspinal** muscles are oriented so their fibers go up and down between the vertebrae (see diagram **m-95**). Contraction of these muscles helps to stabilize, bend, and rotate the spine. Trigger points in these muscles refer pain up and down the spine, into the tailbone, and sometimes to the abdomen and back or inner thigh (see diagram **m-96**). These trigger points are often activated by bending, stooping, and lifting.

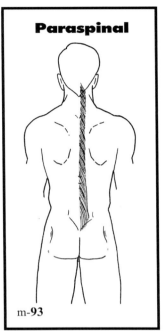

Paraspinal

m-93

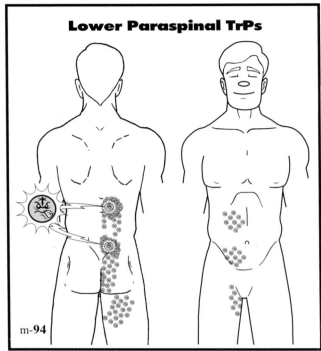

Lower Paraspinal TrPs

m-94

Lower Latissimus

The **lower latissimus** muscle attaches to the top and sides of the pelvic bone (see diagram **m-93**). Contraction of this muscle primarily moves the arm (see page 55). It also helps to stabilize, bend, and rotate the lower spine. Trigger points in this muscle generate pain that can go all the way across the lower back (see diagram **m-94**). These trigger points are often activated by bending, tilting, and twisting the lower spine. This muscle is more likely to cause a pain flair after pushing a vacuum than after pushing a lawn mower.

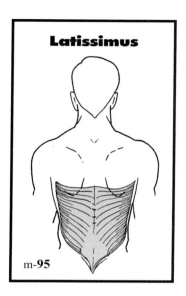

Latissimus

m-**95**

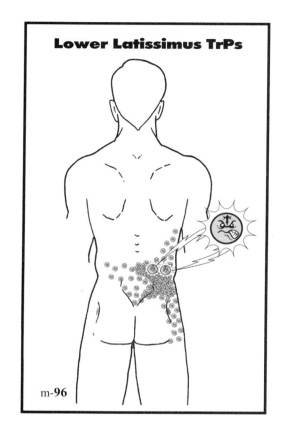

Lower Latissimus TrPs

m-**96**

Rectus Abdominus

The **rectus abdominus** muscle attaches to the lower end of the sternum and front of the lower ribs and inserts across the pubic bone (see diagram **m-97**). It stabilizes the front of the body, flexes the spine, and helps to increase intra-abdominal pressure. Trigger points in the upper part of this muscle can cause abdominal pain, middle back pain, chest pain, and indigestion. Trigger points in the lower part of this muscle may cause abdominal pain, low back pain, and pelvic pain (see diagram **m-98**). The pelvic pain can mimic menstrual cramps. These trigger points are aggravated by chest breathing (without using the diaphragm), overuse and repetitive motion, lifting and twisting activities, and intestinal diseases.

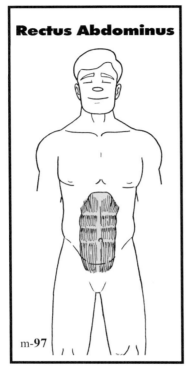

Rectus Abdominus

m-97

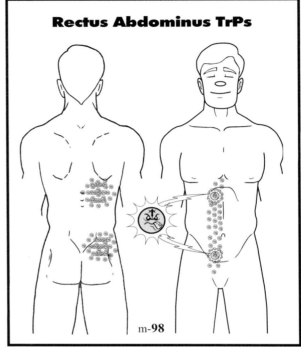

Rectus Abdominus TrPs

m-98

Iliopsoas/Iliacus

The **iliopsoas** muscle attaches to the sides of the lumbar vertebrae and intervertebral discs and inserts on the inside of the upper thigh bone (see diagram **m-99**). The **iliacus** muscle lines the inside of the pelvic bone and joins the iliopsoas where they insert on the inner thigh bone. These connections make this muscle pair a constant stabilizing force for the lower body. They contract during standing, sitting, sit-ups, and flexing the hip (lifting the thigh upwards). Trigger points in this muscle refer pain along the spine of the lower back, into the upper buttocks, and into the front of the thigh and groin (see diagram **m-100**). There may be more pain with weight bearing and less pain with lying down. When these muscles are tight, lying on your back may worsen lower back pain unless there is a pillow placed under your knees.

Sometimes the pain pattern from this muscle pair is more complicated and can contribute to appendicitis or menstrual pain.

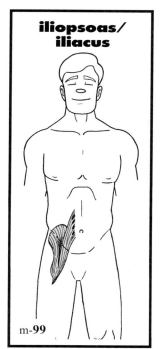

iliopsoas/
iliacus

m-99

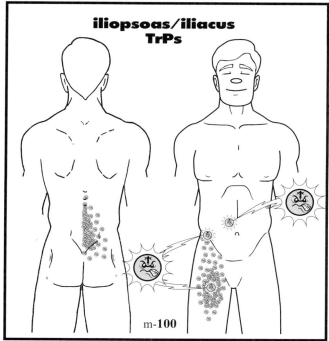

iliopsoas/iliacus
TrPs

m-100

Pelvic Floor

The **pelvic floor** muscles are attached to the coccyx and the back of the pubic bone (not pictured). They control and surround the rectum and sexual organs. They act during bowel, bladder, and sexual functions. The pain pattern from these trigger points can be felt around the tailbone, inner pelvis, groin, and posterior thigh (see diagram **m-101**). These trigger points are also involved in pain patterns sometimes diagnosed as interstitial cystitis or urethral syndrome.

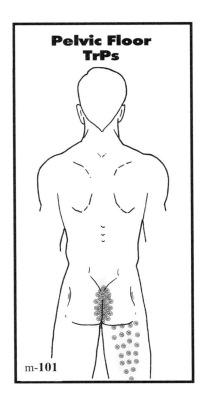

Pelvic Floor TrPs

m-**101**

ABDOMINAL PAIN

Abdominal pain is generated by trigger points in the muscles in the sides and front of the abdomen. These include internal and external obliques, transversus abdominus, and rectus abdominus muscles. These muscles can refer pain to any area of the abdomen and mid to lower back, and may also cause somatovisceral (internal organ) symptoms such as nausea, vomiting, diarrhea, pain with menstruation, or bladder or urinary sphincter spasm. They help to increase intra-abdominal pressure. This stabilizes and strengthens the lower back with lifting activities.

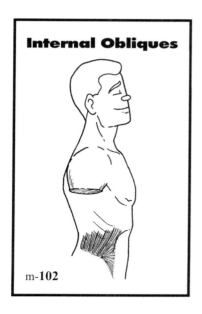

Internal Obliques

m-102

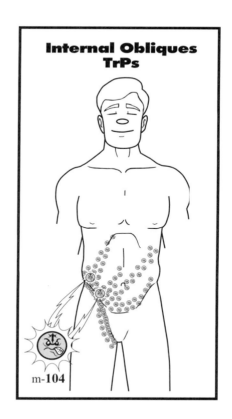

Internal Obliques
TrPs

m-104

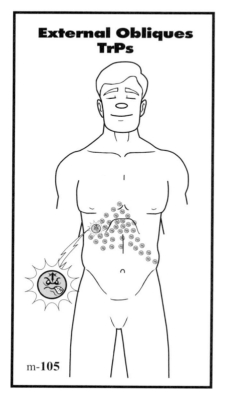

External Obliques
TrPs

m-105

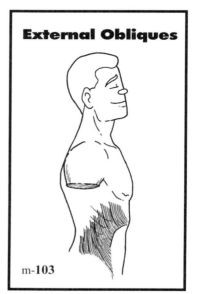

External Obliques

m-103

Internal and External Obliques

The **internal and external oblique** muscles make up the muscular sides of the abdominal wall (see diagrams **m-102** and **m-103**). Contraction of these muscles increases pressure in abdomen and flexes and rotates the spine. Trigger points in these muscles refer pain from the sternum and front of the chest to virtually any part of the abdomen, groin, testicle, or inner thigh (see diagrams **m-104** and **m-105**). They are aggravated by chest breathing (without using the diaphragm), overuse and repetitive motion, lifting and twisting activities, and intestinal diseases.

Rectus Abdominus

The **rectus abdominus** muscle attaches to the lower end of the sternum and front of the lower ribs and inserts across the pubic bone (see diagram

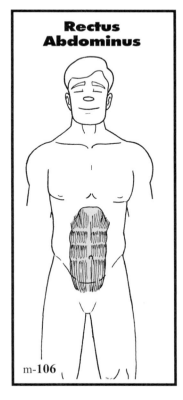

Rectus Abdominus

m-106

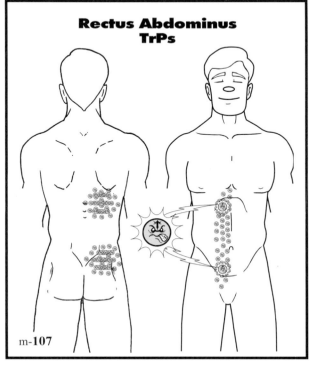

Rectus Abdominus TrPs

m-107

m-106). It stabilizes the front of the body, flexes the spine, and helps to increase intra-abdominal pressure. Trigger points in the upper part of this muscle can cause abdominal pain, middle back pain, chest pain, and indigestion (see diagram **m-107**). Trigger points around the navel may cause pain in the front of the stomach and sensations similar to abdominal cramps. Trigger points in the lower part of this muscle may cause abdominal pain, low back pain, and pelvic pain. The pelvic pain can mimic menstrual cramps. These trigger points are aggravated by breathing without using the diaphragm and intestinal diseases.

PELVIC PAIN

Pelvic pain is generated by trigger points in the many muscles of the pelvic floor, lower back, buttocks, and upper thigh. Refer to those sections to gain a better understanding of pelvic pain. Pelvic floor muscles are not diagrammed. They form the base of the pelvic cavity, going from the pelvic bone to the coccyx.

HIP and BUTTOCKS PAIN

Hip and buttocks pain is generated mostly by trigger points in the muscles that attach at one end or the other to bones of the hip, lower back, and the sides of the thigh. These muscles include the gluteus (maximus, medius, and minimus), piriformis, and tensor fascia lata muscles of the hip. They also include muscles of the lower back and the back and sides of the thigh. The most important trigger points, and the cornerstone for hip pain are in the gluteal and tensor fascia lata muscles. Even though they may be latent and not tender, be sure to include using the ball and stretch techniques on these muscles whenever you are treating pain in the hip area. Orthoses and shoe inserts may be especially helpful in treating hip pain.

Gluteus Maximus

The **gluteus maximus** muscle attaches to the pelvic bone, sacrum, and coccyx, and inserts on the side of the upper thigh bone (see diagram **m-108**).

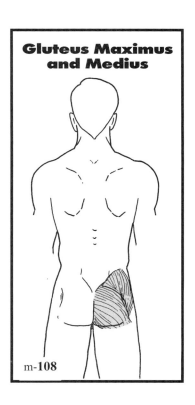

Gluteus Maximus and Medius

m-108

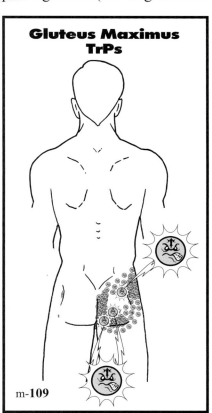

Gluteus Maximus TrPs

m-109

This muscle extends the hip during running, climbing, and jumping. It also assists in maintaining upright posture and outward rotation of the hip. Trigger points in this muscle refer pain through the buttocks, tailbone, and upper posterior thigh (see diagram **m-109**). They will be aggravated by walking uphill or standing with a forward bending posture. Washing dishes at the sink can be especially bothersome.

Gluteus Medius

The **gluteus medius** muscle attaches to the side of the pelvic bone and inserts at the upper side of the thigh bone (see diagram **m-108**). This muscle lifts the thigh out sideways and stabilizes the pelvis when your weight is on one leg as with walking and running. Trigger points in this muscle refer pain to the lower back, sacrum, hip, and outside of the thigh (see diagram **m-110**). They are aggravated by running, jumping, and activities that require standing on one leg (i.e. skating, skiing).

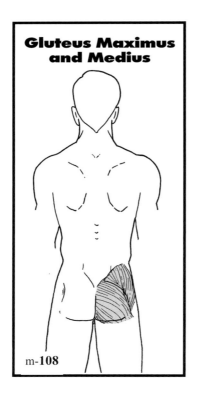

Gluteus Maximus and Medius

m-108

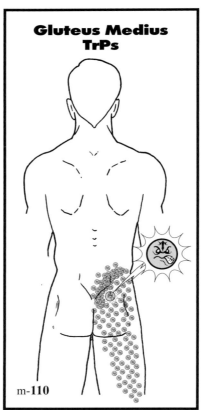

Gluteus Medius TrPs

m-110

Gluteus Minimus

The **gluteus minimus** muscle lies underneath the gluteus medius muscle and has smaller and similar attachments (see diagram **m-111**). It also functions to lift the thigh out sideways and stabilizes the pelvis when your weight is on one leg as with walking and running. Trigger points in this muscle refer pain to the buttocks, hip, posterior thigh, lateral thigh, lateral knee, posterior and lateral calf, and the outside of the ankle (see diagram **m-112**). This pain pattern is often diagnosed as sciatica. These trigger points are aggravated by running, jumping, and activities that require standing on one leg (i.e. skating, skiing).

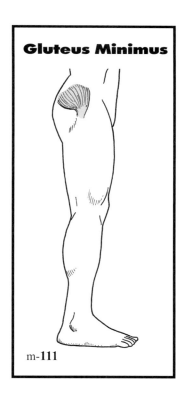

Gluteus Minimus

m-111

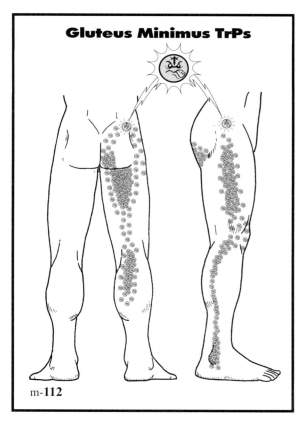

Gluteus Minimus TrPs

m-112

Piriformis

The **piriformis** muscle attaches to the inner aspect of the sacrum, exits the pelvis next to the sciatic nerve, and attaches to the upper aspect of the side of the thigh bone (see diagram **m-113**). This muscle acts primarily to rotate the thigh outwards when the hip is straight. Trigger points in this muscle refer pain across the buttocks, into the hip, and into the upper posterior thigh. These trigger points typically do not refer pain any further down the leg or into the foot (see diagram **m-114**). They can, however, cause muscle tightening that can put pressure on nerve, blood, or lymph vessel. These trigger points are aggravated by running and sitting too long and pushing the gas pedal when driving an automobile.

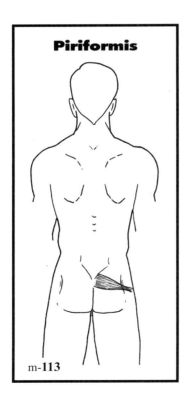

m-113

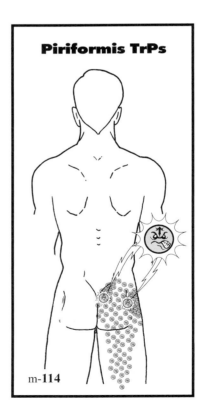

m-114

Tensor Fascia Lata

The **tensor fascia lata** muscle attaches toward the front of the pelvic bone and travels down the outside of the thigh inserting on the outside of the knee and upper calf (see diagram **m-115**). Contraction of this muscle flexes the hip and knee, moves the leg out to the side, and helps stabilize the pelvis when your weight is on one leg as with walking and running. Trigger

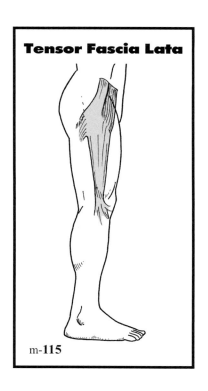

Tensor Fascia Lata

m-115

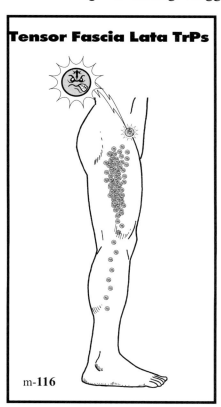

Tensor Fascia Lata TrPs

m-116

points in this muscle refer pain from the waist to the outside of the knee (see diagram **m-116**). Pain from this muscle is likely to radiate to the hip joint and may be misdiagnosed as bursitis. These trigger points are aggravated by running and kicking.

THIGH PAIN

Thigh pain is generated primarily by trigger points in the muscles that move the hip and knee joints. Lower back, pelvic floor and calf muscles can also refer pain to various areas of the thigh. Thigh muscles can generally be divided into four groups, based upon their location around the thigh bone (outside, front, inside, and back). The tensor fascia lata is located along the outside of the thigh. The sartorius and quadriceps are located in the front of the thigh. The quadriceps is a group of four muscles that include the vastus lateralis, rectus femoris, vastus intermedius, and vastus medialis. The adductor muscles are located along the inside of the thigh. Adductors include the adductor longus, adductor brevis, adductor magnus, pectineus, and gracilis. Hamstring muscles are located along the back of the thigh. Treating hamstring muscles is especially important for reducing lower back pain. Latent trigger points cause the hamstrings to remain tight, resulting in increased lower back stress with walking. Treating quadriceps muscles is especially important for treating knee pain. Orthoses and shoe inserts may be especially helpful in treating thigh pain.

Tensor Fascia Lata

The **tensor fascia lata** muscle attaches toward the front of the pelvic bone and travels down the outside of the thigh inserting on the outside of the knee and upper calf (see diagram **m-115**). Contraction of this muscle flexes the hip and knee, moves the leg out to the side, and helps stabilize the pelvis when your weight is on one leg as with walking and running. Trigger points in this muscle refer pain from the waist to the outside of the knee (see diagram **m-116**). Pain from this muscle is likely to radiate to the hip joint and may be misdiagnosed as bursitis. These trigger points are aggravated by running and kicking.

Quadriceps and Sartorius

The **quadriceps** muscle group (vastus medialis, vastus lateralis, vastus intermedius, and rectus femoris) attaches to the front of the upper thigh, except the rectus femoris which attaches to the front of the lower pelvis. These four muscles then join, envelope the knee cap, and insert on the front of the upper shin (see diagram **m-117**). Their basic function is to straighten the knee joint. The rectus femoris also helps to flex the hip joint. Trigger points in this muscle group may refer pain, numbness, tingling, or burning along the front, inside, and outside of the thigh from the hip to the knee (see diagrams **m-118**, **m-119** and **m-120**). These

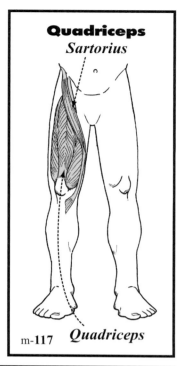

Quadriceps
Sartorius

m-117   *Quadriceps*

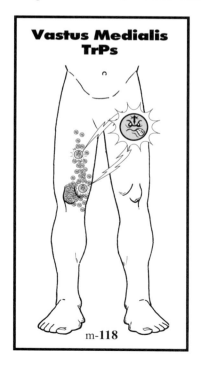

Vastus Medialis TrPs

m-118

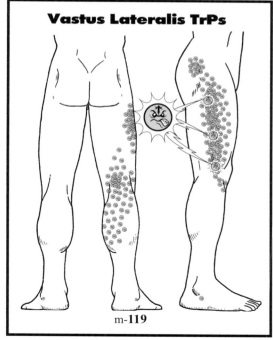

Vastus Lateralis TrPs

m-119

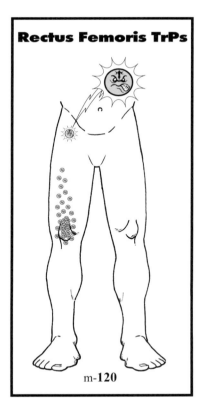

Rectus Femoris TrPs

m-**120**

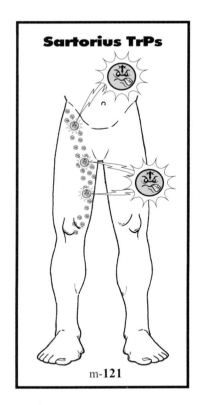

Sartorius TrPs

m-**121**

trigger points can also cause pain in the knee joint (see diagrams **m-118** and **m-120**). The outside part of the quadriceps (vastus lateralis) can refer pain below the knee to the back and side of the calf (see diagram **m-119**). The vastus intermedius pain pattern is similar to the other diagrammed quadriceps muscles and is not shown separately.

The **sartorius** muscle attaches to the upper outer pelvis and to the inside of the upper shin. Its function is to assist with hip and knee flexion. Trigger points in this muscle cause a pain pattern that is localized more to the front of the thigh (see diagram **m-121**).

Among the more remarkable symptoms caused by trigger points in these muscles (quadriceps and sartorius) are numbness and tingling over the front of the thigh (see diagrams **m-118**, **m-120**, and **m-121**). The numbness can be constant or intermittent and it is not necessarily associated with pain. In addition, the numbness and tingling generated by these trigger points are likely to cross to the other thigh. Indeed, this altered sensation in either thigh is likely to be caused by active or latent trigger points in both thighs simultaneously. Treating either thigh alone is likely to result in significant improvement in both thighs.

Trigger points in these muscles are aggravated by running, climbing, jumping, kneeling, and abnormalities with the motion of walking (gait).

Hip Adductors

The **adductor** muscles (adductor longus, adductor brevis, adductor magnus, pectineus, and gracilis) attach to the pubic and buttocks bones and insert along the inside of the thigh bone, almost as far down as the knee (see diagram **m-122**). Contraction of these muscles brings the knees together, closing the legs. Trigger points in these muscles refer pain to the groin, front of the hip, knee, and along the inside and front of the thigh and lower leg

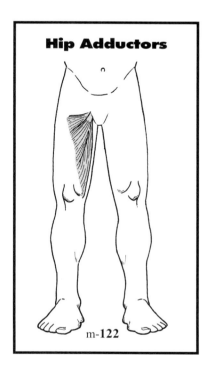

m-122

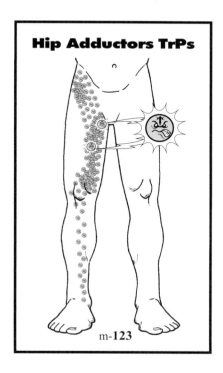

m-123

(see diagram **m-123**). They are especially aggravated by holding the knees together and walking on a slippery surface.

Hamstrings

The **hamstring** muscles (biceps femoris, semitendinosus, semimembranosus) attach to the buttocks bone and insert on the leg bones behind and past the knee (see diagram **m-124**). Contraction of these muscles bends the

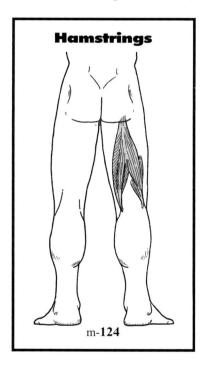

m-**124**

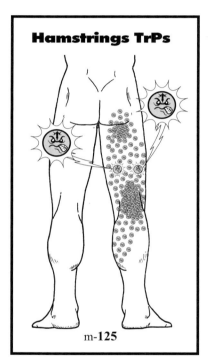

m-**125**

knee and assists with extending the hip. Trigger points in these muscles refer pain along the back of the leg from the buttocks to the calf (see diagram **m-125**). They may also refer pain to the back of the knee joint. These trigger points are aggravated by walking and running.

CALF and LOWER LEG PAIN

Pain in the calf and lower leg is generated primarily by trigger points in the muscles that move the knee, ankle, and toe joints. It can also be caused by muscles that move the hip joint. Muscles in the front of the leg include tibialis anterior and the toe extensors. Muscles in the back of the leg include gastrocnemius, tibialis posterior, soleus, and the toe flexors. Muscles along the outside of the leg include peroneus longus, brevis, and tertius. Treating these muscles is important for reducing ankle, foot, and toe pain. Muscles along the side and in the back of the leg are often involved in causing the pain of plantar fascitis. Orthoses and shoe inserts may be especially helpful in treating calf and foot pain.

Tibialis Anterior and Toe Extensors

Tibialis anterior and **toe extensor** muscles attach to the front of the leg and the top of the foot and toes. They act to bend the ankle upwards and

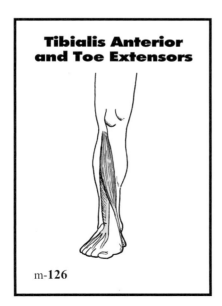

Tibialis Anterior and Toe Extensors

m-126

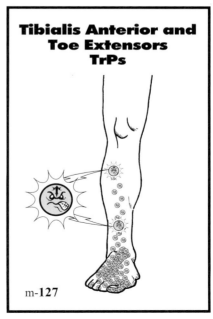

Tibialis Anterior and Toe Extensors TrPs

m-127

94

raise the toes (see diagram **m-126**). Trigger points in these muscles refer pain to the front of the shin, top of the ankle and foot, and to the toes (see diagram **m-127**). They may cause the pain known as "shin splints" and they may also cause severe pain in the great toe. These trigger points are aggravated by running.

Gastrocnemius, Tibialis Posterior, and Soleus

The **gastrocnemius** muscles attach to the back of the thigh near the knee joint and also to the back of the heel. The **tibialis posterior** (not shown separately) and **soleus** muscles attach to the back of the calf near the knee joint and also to the back of the heel (see diagram **m-128** and **m-130**). These muscles act primarily to push the foot down. The gastrocnemius muscles

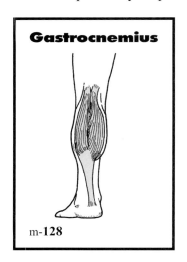

m-**128**

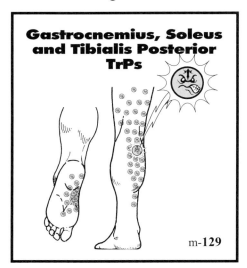

m-**129**

also assist with bending the knee. Trigger points in these muscles cause pain in the back of the thigh, knee, calf, heel cord, heel, and ankle (see diagram **m-129**). They may also cause severe pain in the bottom of the foot. This pain may be misdiagnosed as coming from a heel spur or plantar fascitis. Calf cramps are often caused by trigger points in these muscles. Sometimes these cramps are most noticeable at night and awaken people from sleep.

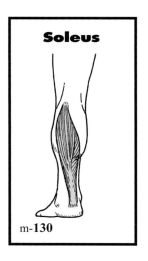

Soleus

m-**130**

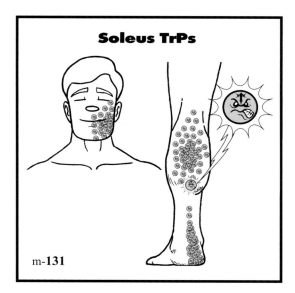

Soleus TrPs

m-**131**

Soleus muscle trigger points can also cause pain in the same side of the face and jaw (see diagram **m-131**). **Phantom limb pain** in an amputated leg or foot is often caused by trigger points in these muscles. Trigger points in these muscles are aggravated by walking, running, and jumping.

Toe Flexors

The **toe flexor** muscles lie underneath the gastrocnemius and soleus muscles, attaching to the back of the calf and the underside of the toe bones (see diagram **m-128** and **m-130**). Toe flexors are not diagramed separately. Contraction of these muscles curls the toes. Trigger points in these muscles refer pain to the inside of the lower leg, the bottom of the foot, and the great toe (see diagram **m-132**). They are aggravated by walking and running.

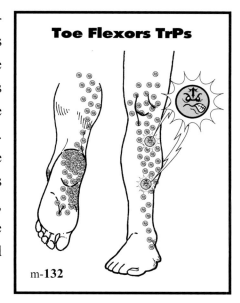

Toe Flexors TrPs

m-**132**

Peroneus (Longus, Brevis, Tertius)

The **peroneus** muscles attach to the outside of the leg below the knee and also to the outside of the foot (see diagram **m-133**). They act to bend the ankle outwards and assist with flexing the ankle. Trigger points in these muscles refer pain primarily to the outside of the lower leg, ankle, and foot

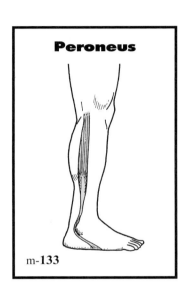

Peroneus

m-133

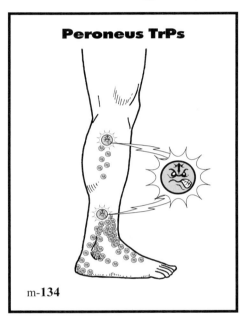

Peroneus TrPs

m-134

(see diagram **m-134**). They are especially important in treating plantar fascitis. These trigger points are aggravated by walking, running, jumping, and poor foot wear.

Toe Extensors

The **toe extensor** muscles lie underneath the peroneus muscles, attaching to the front and outside of the leg below the knee, and to the tops of the toes (see diagram **m-135**). They act to straighten the toes. The pain pattern from these trigger points is primarily localized to the top of the foot (see diagram **m-136**). These trigger points are aggravated by walking, running, and poor foot wear.

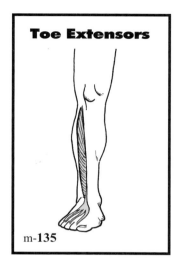

Toe Extensors

m-135

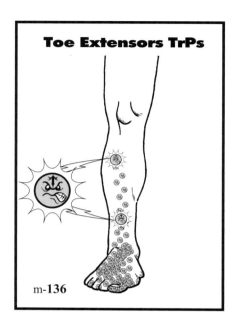

Toe Extensors TrPs

m-136

FOOT PAIN

Pain in the foot is generated primarily by trigger points in muscles of the calf, lower leg (discussed previously), and foot. Muscles of the foot serve chiefly to move the toes. They are located mostly underneath and between the bones in the middle of the foot. These muscles are often involved in causing foot cramps and some of the pain of plantar fascitis.

Top of the Foot

Muscles along the **top of the foot** attach to the foot bones and the top of the toe bones (see diagram **m-137**). They act to extend the toes. Trigger points in these muscles refer pain to the top of the foot (see diagram **m-138**). They may also cause pain misdiagnosed as Morton's neuroma.

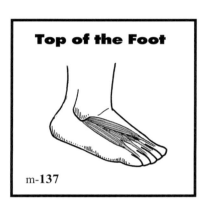

Top of the Foot

m-137

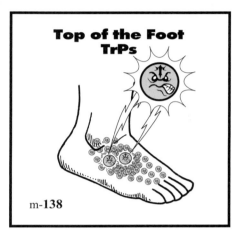

Top of the Foot TrPs

m-138

Bottom of the foot

Muscles on the **bottom of the foot** attach to the foot bones and the underside of the toe bones (see diagram **m-139**). They act primarily to curl the toes. Trigger points in these muscles refer pain along the inside of the

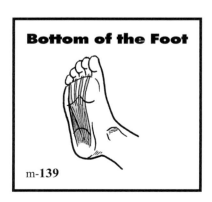

Bottom of the Foot

m-139

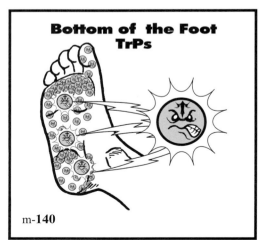

Bottom of the Foot TrPs

m-140

foot and heel, under the foot, and under the toes (see diagram **m-140**). These pain patterns are often misdiagnosed as plantar fascitis and heel spurs. Pain from these trigger points may also be misdiagnosed as bunion pain and Morton's neuroma.

ball massage
chapter

ball massage

Your Best Friend Is A...

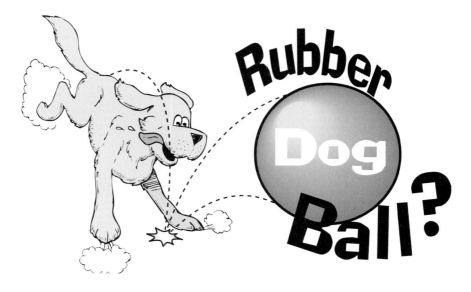

It is a wonderful idea to massage your body at least once per day. Massage increases blood flow to the muscles, facilitates the removal of toxins, and reduces the activity of myofascial trigger points.

Usually, your extremities (arms, legs, hands, and feet) can be reached and easily massaged using your hands. Your back and buttocks, however, are best reached with a ball. In addition, if your hands lack the strength to massage the places they can reach, a ball can be used to massage almost anywhere. Tennis balls are a great size for most areas of the body and are readily available, though we have found from personal experience that hard rubber balls are easier to use. Thinner people with more fragile pain conditions may prefer softer balls from the toy store.

Deeper work and a firmer massage can be achieved with a rubber "dog" ball or lacrosse ball. It is also worthwhile to experiment with racket balls and squash balls. Each person is different and balls come in many sizes. Try several and see what you like for each area of your body.

General Principles

The ball is basically used in two ways: to generally massage all of the tissue in an area or to apply pressure to specific trigger points. General massage will enhance blood flow and remove toxins from the muscle. Pressure to specific trigger points will make them smaller. When trigger points are smaller, they generate less pain.

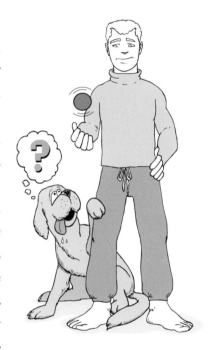

One of the reasons for stiffness and soreness in the body is that the muscles are tighter than they need to be. When muscles are tighter, they use more energy. The tightness of the muscle, however, prevents the much needed increase in blood flow and nutrient supply. Another effect of the decreased blood flow is that "exhaust" from the muscles cannot be carried away as effectively. As a result, the muscles are "holding their breath" and they are "full of toxic stuff."

Myofascial pain is always generated by multiple knots (trigger points) in several related muscles. Active and latent trigger points send impulses to the brain that are interpreted as a pain pattern. Even a localized pain pattern is generated by several trigger points in more than one muscle. While it may be quite satisfying to apply pressure to only the most tender trigger point or to the most painful area, more lasting relief may be achieved by massaging all of the trigger points involved in the pain pattern.

To massage all of the trigger points and improve blood flow to the muscle, use the ball in a method similar to mowing the lawn. Simply roll over each part of the muscle moving the ball up and down or sideways. Try to roll once over each part of the muscle, and do not work long on any one area. Rolling over each area just once is quite sufficient to "give the muscle a breath." Breathing and relaxing during this technique are not very important, and the exercise can be done when under stress or in a hurry.

Start gently, and just briefly "dust" your muscles with the massage technique. Be sure to drink lots of water to help your body eliminate the toxins that will be set free. Once you are more coordinated and stop dropping the ball, massage from the neck to the buttocks can be done in one or two minutes.

When the ball is being used to apply pressure to one specific trigger point at a time, start with gentle pressure and then gradually increase the pressure or move slowly to "follow" the trigger point's maximum pain site. Breathing and relaxation are of the utmost importance when using the ball in this fashion to "melt" a trigger point.

THE TORSO

Neck

The muscles along the back of the neck can be massaged using ball techniques. Hair needs to be pulled up and out of the way as it can easily caught up by the ball and pulled out at the roots. The best position is usually standing with the back to the wall (see diagram **b-1**). Place the ball at the back of the neck, just to one side and not directly over the spine. With a slight bending and straightening of the knees, the body will move up and down, allowing the ball to massage the muscles in the back of the neck. Allow the upper back to rub against the wall. The hips may need to be several inches

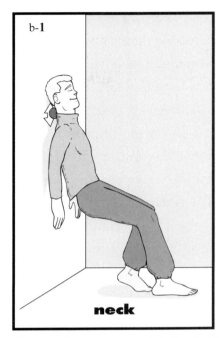

b-1

neck

from the wall for the neck to make contact with the ball. Do not massage the middle of the neck where the spine bones can be felt (it is uncomfortable and doesn't help to loosen and massage the paraspinal muscles). There is no need to apply more than gentle pressure, and a few passes will usually be sufficient. Repeat this technique for the other side. The muscles on the side of the neck cannot be reached using these techniques, and **the front of the neck should never be massaged** (the windpipe and carotid arteries could be damaged).

Mid/Upper Back

The mid/upper back is divided into three areas: between the shoulder blades, the shoulder blades specifically, and the upper shoulders. It is important to work on and loosen all three areas for relief of mid to upper back pain and headache.

The middle back is worked on with an up and down motion as the ball is rolled on each side between the spine and the shoulder blades (see diagram

b-2). It is easiest to start with the back and buttocks touching the wall. Then the upper body is leaned forward and the ball is dropped over one shoulder. With the buttocks still resting against the wall, the upper body is slowly leaned forward and the ball is lowered to be level with the bottom of the shoulder blades. The feet are then moved forward a little further away from the wall, the buttocks are lifted off the wall, and pressure is applied to the ball. By flexing and extending the hips and knees, the ball will massage the mid/upper back including the middle trapezius, rhomboid, and paraspinal muscles.

If performing this technique bothers your knees or you have too much difficulty controlling the ball, there is a simpler technique. Put the ball in a stocking and lower it over your shoulder behind you. Instead of flexing your hips and knees to raise and lower your body, slightly rotate back and forth so that the ball moves sideways between your spine and shoulder blade. Work only one side at a time and **do not** roll the ball over the spine bones. Raise and lower the stocking/ball so that you can massage from your upper to lower back.

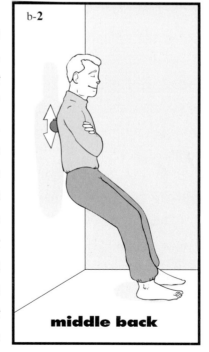

b-2

middle back

A quicker technique that may require more practice is to "limbo" with the ball. After lowering it to the level of mid-shoulder blade, move your heels approximately 12-17 inches from the wall you are leaning against. Then simply move your belly out away from the wall and then back towards the wall. Do not think about bending your knees. Just the motion of "belly out-belly in" will make the ball massage the area from the shoulder blade to the top of the shoulder. The best arm position for this technique is to cross both arms over your chest and tuck your hands in so that your shoulders and arms can be restful.

Pain symptoms next to the shoulder blade are always partly caused by a group of trigger points located in the muscles that are directly over the shoulder blade itself. To massage these areas, turn 45 degrees toward the wall, cross both arms over the chest, tuck in the hands, and place the ball directly over the shoulder blade (see diagram **b-3**). With the arms crossed and the hands tucked in, the shoulders can be more relaxed and the hips and shoulders will rotate together during this exercise. If the arms are hanging by the sides, there will be more twisting at the waist and your shoulders will be more tense.

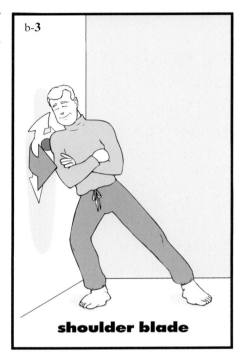

b-3

shoulder blade

Once in this position, begin rotating the body so that the ball rolls over the shoulder blade and the side of the body under the back of the arm. Do not roll off the back of the shoulder blade towards the spine. As this gentle twisting motion is performed, slowly flex and extend the hips and knees so that the body is lowered and raised and the ball covers an area from the upper to the lower shoulder blade. Make the knee bend much slower than the twisting, and only go down and up once or twice. The muscles massaged by this technique include the infraspinatus, upper latissimus, and teres.

The upper shoulder is best worked on in a seated position, leaning backwards with the buttocks several inches away from the wall. Place the ball behind the upper shoulder and rest the head against the wall (see diagram **b-4**). Let the ball push on a "good spot" and just relax and take a

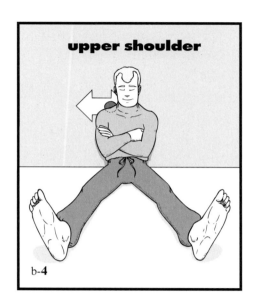

few deep breaths. With relaxation and gentle pressure, the shoulder trapezius and levator scapulae muscles will relax. The upper body can be gently moved slightly sideways where another "good spot" can usually be discovered. The best position for the arms is crossed in front and resting across the chest. This reduces the weight held by the shoulders, and they will relax more deeply.

There is another very powerful technique for using the ball to ease upper back and neck pain. This technique can be uncomfortable and painful, but it is worth the trouble. The discomfort should be at a low enough level that full relaxation can be achieved.

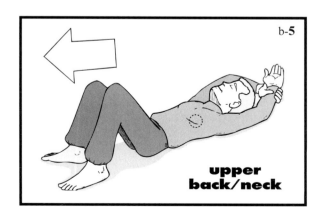

The technique is performed while lying on the back on a bed or cushioned mat (see diagram **b-5**). Place the ball to the side of the spine at about the level of the lower part of the shoulder blade and allow the mind and body to relax. Next, raise the arm on the same side as the ball up above the head with the hand resting on the mattress. Hold this wrist with the other hand, and gently pull the wrist upward and toward the side of the holding arm. Relax the body and the ball will seem to work into the muscles under the shoulder blade. Then, gradually scoot the entire body in the direction of the feet, an inch or so at a time. With each scoot, another painful spot will be encountered. Pause at each spot to relax and let the muscle release. Continue to move the body in the direction of the feet and the ball will move upward to the top of the shoulder. Repeat this technique on the other side of the back. As this technique is performed, pain may radiate to the neck, head, and jaw. The neck and upper body will usually feel much looser after this exercise.

Lower Back

Lower back pain comes mainly from muscles in the lower back and buttocks (see Lower Extremities section for buttocks massage technique). The lower back is worked with the ball in two basic positions: standing and lying down.

In the standing position, the ball is placed to the side of the spine in the small of the lower back (see diagram **b-6**). The feet are moved away from the wall and the hips and knees are flexed and extended to create an up and down massaging action with the ball. A gentle sideways motion will ensure coverage of a wider area, but **be careful not**

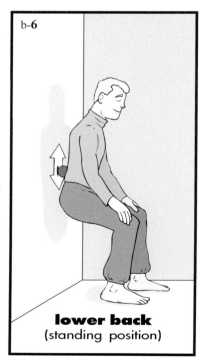

b-6

lower back
(standing position)

to roll the ball directly over the spine, as that is generally uncomfortable and not helpful.

In the lying down position, place the ball next to the spine, above the pelvic bone, and below the ribs (see diagram **b-7**). Raise the knees and rest the feet flat on the floor. As the body relaxes, the ball will "sink into" and soften the paraspinal muscles of the lower back. The hands can rest comfortably on the abdomen (not shown). Next, slowly scoot the body an inch towards the head and then towards the feet. Pain may shoot up the back or down into the buttocks and leg as pressure is applied to the trigger points in these muscles. The lower back will be looser afterwards.

The lower back muscles can also be massaged in this position by moving the body up and down towards the head and then towards the feet. To make this motion easier, "unweight" the shoulders and upper back by placing the hands on the floor above the shoulders and lifting.

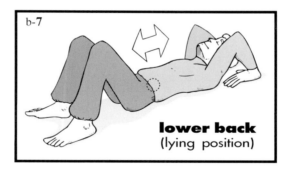

b-7

lower back
(lying position)

Chest

When the upper back area is tight and painful, the upper chest and pectoralis musculature is also usually tight. Working on this area of the body will help the upper back to soften. Loosening the front of the chest will also allow chest expansion and promote better posture with less tendency for the shoulders to roll forward.

To perform this technique, face towards the wall and place the ball

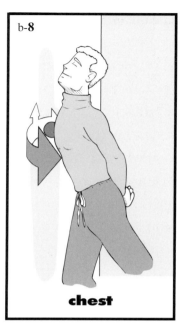

chest

under the collarbone (clavicle), and above the breast tissue (see diagram **b-8**). Keeping the neck relaxed, turn the face toward the opposite shoulder. Place the arms behind the back and clasp the hands. Relax the shoulders, chest, and hands while gently rocking back and forth sideways. Always remember to work on both sides during each session. When switching to the other side lift off the ball; **do not** roll over the breast bone.

UPPER EXTREMITIES

The arms, forearms, and even the hands can be massaged using ball techniques. In general, parts of the body that are further away from the center have nerves and arteries closer to the skin. It is conceivable that these **structures can be injured if too much pressure is applied**. The median nerve runs along the inside of the upper arm beneath the biceps muscle, through the front of the elbow, and then along the middle of the forearm to cross the palm side of the wrist. The ulnar nerve travels down the upper arm, around the inside of the elbow to the fingers, and then through the little finger side of the wrist. The "funny bone" is where this nerve crosses the elbow. Hitting this nerve at the elbow causes a weird tingling and burning sensation that shoots to the hand and fingers. Arteries to the hand are under the middle of the palm. Massaging these areas and structures too roughly can cause injury. Numbness can occur from a pressure injury to a nerve. Too much pressure over an artery can also be damaging and is discouraged. If the ball massage techniques are applied with caution, any such unfavorable symptoms should be temporary and quickly reversible. Properly applied, firm pressure over muscles and trigger points will be rewarding. These techniques can help relieve a wide variety of pains in the upper extremities, including the symptoms associated with tennis elbow and carpal tunnel syndrome.

Biceps

The biceps muscle is difficult to massage using ball techniques. This technique requires a twisting force that must be supported by the chest and abdominal muscles while flexing and extending the knees and hips to move the body up and down (see diagram **b-9**).

In performing this ball technique, the arm can be positioned across the front of the body, hanging down from the shoulder (not shown). This will minimize the twisting forces needed by the body's trunk. The arm can also be positioned next to the body, but the twisting forces are accentuated with this positioning.

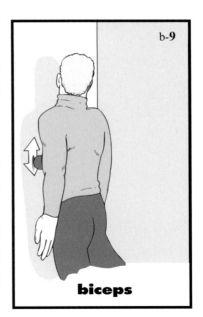

b-**9**

biceps

Triceps

The triceps muscle is relatively easy to massage using the ball techniques. It can be worked on in a standing (see diagram **b-10**) or seated position (see

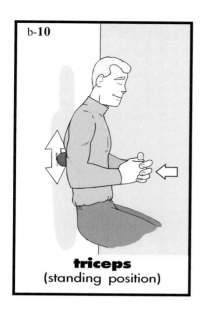

triceps
(standing position)

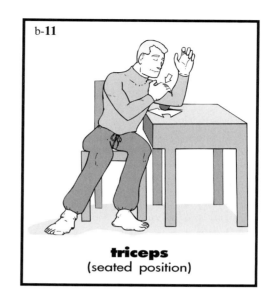

triceps
(seated position)

diagram **b-11**). In either position, place the ball behind or under the triceps muscle. Then move the arm in such a manner that the muscle is massaged along its length. *In a standing posture*, the opposite hand should contribute much of the backwards directed force so that the upper back muscles can be relaxed. *In a seated position*, the opposite hand can apply a downward directed force over the biceps (see diagram **b-11**). The opposite hand can also stabilize the arm over the ball so the shoulder muscles can be more relaxed.

Forearm

If you imagine the length of the forearm divided into thirds, most of the forearm's muscle mass is located in the third closest to the elbow. Generally, massage techniques should be applied to this area of muscle and *not to the areas near the wrist where ligaments and nerves are close to the surface of the skin and can be injured*. Trigger points in these muscles can be treated with massage techniques to the palm side or conversely to the top side of the forearm. Muscles of the forearm refer pain to the elbow, wrist, and finger areas.

Golfer's elbow is one example of pain located on the inner side of the elbow. Trigger points for this area can be massaged in a seated position with the ball placed between the palm side of the forearm and a table (see diagram **b-12**). Apply gentle pressure downwards with the opposite hand while slowly moving the massaged forearm so that the ball travels from the elbow towards the wrist and back again. **Do not** use the muscles under the shoulder of the massaged arm to pull it down towards the

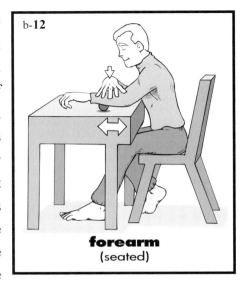

forearm
(seated)

table and **do not** apply a lot of pressure with the other hand during this technique. The ulnar nerve is usually located within these tissues and pressure may produce a sensation similar to hitting the "funny bone."

Tennis elbow is one example of pain located on the outer side of the elbow. Trigger points for this area are best massaged in a standing position

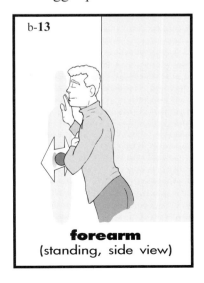

forearm
(standing, side view)

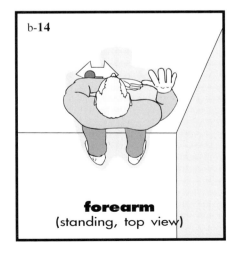

forearm
(standing, top view)

with the elbow bent approximately 90 degrees and resting against the abdomen (see diagram **b-13** and **b-14**). Place the ball between the top side of the forearm and a wall, lean slightly towards the wall, and allow the body weight to apply gentle pressure against the ball. Slowly rock sideways back and forth so that the ball moves along the forearm from the elbow towards the wrist area (see diagram **b-14**). This technique should be gentle. **Do not** apply ball pressure to the bone of the elbow as this will be uncomfortable and not productive.

Hand

Most muscular hand pain is caused by myofascial trigger points in the large group of muscles located between the thumb and index finger. This area can be massaged using a ball the size of a handball or a small dog ball. Place the ball on a table, the massaged hand over the ball, and the opposite hand on top (see diagram **b-15** and **b-16**). Use a gentle combination of

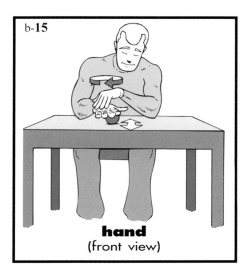

b-15

hand
(front view)

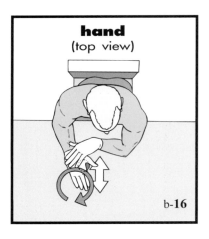

hand
(top view)

b-16

circular and back and forth motions to work on these muscles while applying a small amount of pressure with the opposite hand. **Do not** be overly forceful because there are nerves and blood vessels that can be damaged if they are pinched between the ball and the hand bones.

LOWER EXTREMITIES

Buttock/Hamstring

The upper buttocks is best massaged in an upright position and leaning against a wall. Stand comfortably near the wall with the body rotated approximately 45 degrees and the feet placed under the shoulders and slightly out from the wall (see diagram **b-17**). Cross both arms and tuck in the hands so that the shoulders can be totally relaxed while the forearms lay across the chest. The ball is placed over the upper-outer portion of the buttocks and then the entire torso (shoulders to hips) is rotated in both directions as the ball massages the upper buttocks from the back to the side of the hip area. **Do not** massage or rub on the S-I (sacroiliac) joint. This is uncomfortable and not generally helpful.

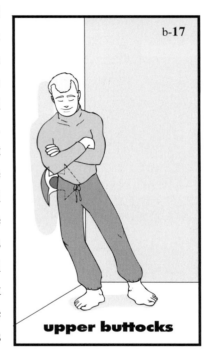

b-17

upper buttocks

The S-I joints are located above and to each side of the tail bone.

The massage is performed by rotating the body left and right, thereby covering the area from the back of the buttocks to the outer hip. As the body is rotated, slowly flex the knees and hips so that the body is lowered to massage the upper hip, and then straighten so that the ball massages lower over the hip and buttocks.

The lower buttocks and upper hamstring massage can be done in a hallway or a place where it is possible to be sandwiched between two parallel walls. Stand with the back against one wall and then lean forward until it is possible to brace the arms against the opposite wall. Place the ball directly behind the buttock and lean against it so that the body weight is balanced upon the ball (see diagram **b-18**). Rotate the body sideways back and forth so that the ball covers as much of the lower buttocks as comfortably possible. Flexing the hips and knees to lower the body and raising up a little on the toes will allow for more of the area to be massaged. It is not unusual to feel pain shooting up to the lower back or down the leg while these techniques are being performed.

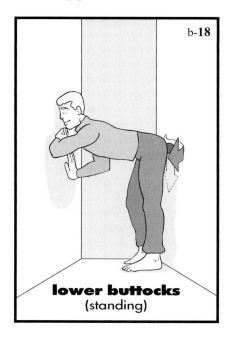

b-18

lower buttocks
(standing)

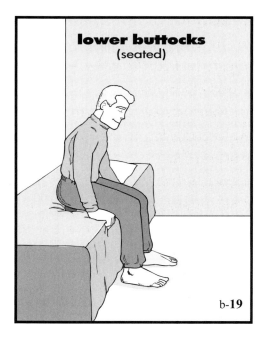

lower buttocks
(seated)

b-19

Another technique for massaging this area is to sit near the edge of a mattress with the ball placed under the buttocks or upper thigh (see diagram **b-19**). Use the hands to support some of the body weight and then move the body front/back, sideways, or in circles to massage the area. If more pressure is needed, this technique can be performed on a slightly cushioned chair.

Calf/Hamstring

Calf and hamstring musculature trigger points can be massaged in seated or standing positions. In a seated position, place the ball under the calf (thigh for hamstrings) and apply pressure to a tender trigger point (see diagram **b-20**). Take some slow breaths for relaxation and allow the muscle to soften. The ball can be moved and placed under other areas of the muscle as needed.

b-20

calf
(seated position)

Calf and hamstring massage in a standing position is easier to perform holding on to some support. In a standing position with the back to a wall, place the ball behind the thigh and lean into it (see diagram **b-21**). Up and down massage can be performed in a limited fashion by flexing the ankles. The muscle fibers can also be cross-massaged by using a gentle sideways motion.

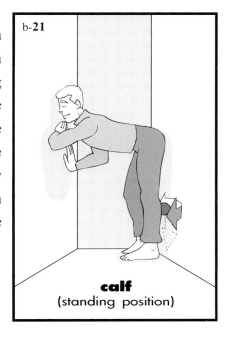

b-**21**

calf
(standing position)

Foot

Foot and heel pain is often caused by myofascial trigger points in the muscles underneath the foot. These can be massaged using a ball the size of a handball or small dog ball (see diagram **b-22**). Sit with the feet on the floor. Place the ball under one foot and massage the muscles with a combination of circular and front-to-back motions. This technique does not require much pressure. For the most part, enough pressure can be applied by the weight of the leg. If additional pressure is needed, place a hand on the thigh or lean forward and rest a forearm upon the thigh.

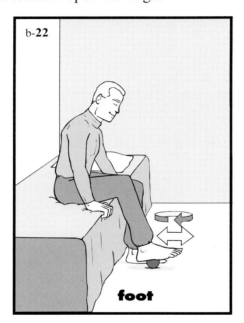

b-22

foot

ball

stretching
chapter

stretching
part 1
GENERAL PRINCIPLES OF STRETCHING

Most People Have Been Taught...

Most people with a history of chronic pain have had some experience with stretching in physical therapy, yoga, or relaxation classes. Regardless of your background, this is perhaps the most important section to read and understand. At whatever level a person's ability lies, there is always room to grow and have these skills become more effective.

Real Stretch Happens in the Mind

There are five basic principles that need to be understood with regard to stretching virtually any muscle in the body.

The first is that **real stretch happens in the mind**. This cannot be over-emphasized. Keep the forces very gentle, and **do not** try to force the body to stretch with pulling and pushing. We are trying to stretch the trigger points in the muscle and their fascia. These trigger points

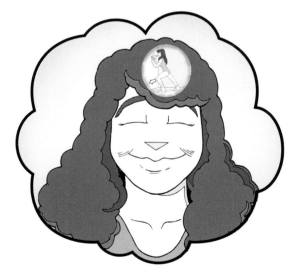

the real stretch happens in your mind...

are held by the sympathetic nervous system and they will not stretch by pulling on the ends of the muscle. Pulling on the muscle to make it longer will only stretch the normal and weaker muscle fibers. In fact, when forceful stretching lengthens the normal muscle, the trigger points may "seize" the extra slack and tighten even more. This will result in the stretching exercise causing more pain. If you have had a previous stretching experience that subsequently caused more pain, it is even more important to understand this concept so that the next experience is more favorable.

Use breath as a tool to relax the body and the mind, thereby allowing the stretch to occur. Then, when the body moves to look like it is stretching, only move enough to "take up the slack" that was created by the relaxation/breathing.

Second, **do not stretch into pain**. Stretching does not have to be comfortable, but it should not be painful. Real stretch is all about relaxation, and pain from stretching makes relaxation unnecessarily difficult.

Third, how far the muscle stretches is not an important goal. The immediate **objective of stretching should be to make the muscle looser, not to make the body move farther**. Success in stretching has very little to do with how far the body moves. Even people with a normal neck range of motion can have tight muscles and myofascial neck pain. These people will not generally move further after stretching. Most of the time, if you focus on getting the mind and muscles to relax, the muscles will soften and more motion will occur.

The fourth basic principle is that stretching must be performed **very slowly and gently**. Indeed, the slower and more gently the body is moved, the more effective the stretch will be.

Lastly, the **body is like a rubber band in that a stretched muscle goes back to being tight**. If you keep a rubber band stretched out for a few weeks, however, it will not return to its previous length. In a similar fashion, periodically stretch the muscle throughout the day to prevent it from fully retightening (see pages 130-131).

Down-Regulating the Sympathetic Nervous System

The sympathetic nervous system was discussed previously (see page 26). The quickest way to increase activity and cause a reaction with respect to the sympathetic nervous system is to suddenly place yourself in a situation of utmost stress. Activation of the sympathetic nervous system will cause increased heart rate, respiration rate, and sweating. When the sympathetic nervous system is activated, it also causes tightening of the body's trigger points and this causes pain to increase. The quickest way to decrease the activity of the sympathetic nervous system is with relaxation. As the mind relaxes, the muscles become limp, and real stretch becomes possible.

Breathing is the Easiest Tool to Learn

Breathing is the easiest tool to learn in order to facilitate the relaxation that makes stretching more successful. There are as many ways of developing these techniques as there are people who use them. As you practice and develop the breathing techniques for this work, keep in mind that the goal is to facilitate relaxation. Relaxation occurs best as air is breathed out of the body.

To further understand this

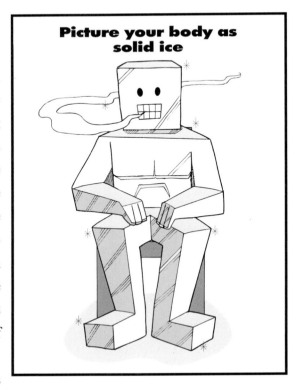

Picture your body as solid ice

stretch

123

idea, imagine your body as being made of solid ice, rigid and unyielding. As you slowly exhale, you should try to feel your body melting to the floor. Your body should feel like it is being transformed from an icy block into a loose and flowing liquid. The more completely your mind allows your body to experience this sensation, the better and deeper your stretches will be.

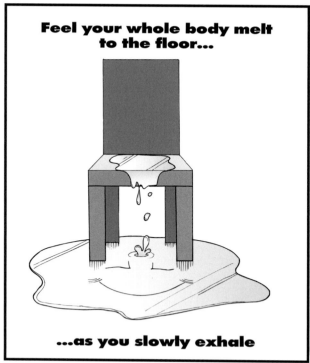

Feel your whole body melt to the floor...

...as you slowly exhale

It is not important to take a deep breath. In fact, it is often better if the breath is not very deep. More shallow breathing is especially important when the muscles being stretched are in the upper body. This is because the muscles used for breath include those in the upper shoulders and neck, and they cannot relax as well if they are working hard at breathing. Try to keep these muscles and the shoulders as calm as possible during the breathing for all stretching.

It is best to inhale using the diaphragm. Diaphragmatic breathing will cause the stomach area of the body to move out with inhalation and in with exhalation. If the diaphragm does most of the work, the upper shoulders and chest can remain still. The less these muscles work with this breathing, the better the technique and the more effective the relaxation. The breath should not be deep enough to cause the shoulders to rise or tension to be increased in the upper body.

Breathing Technique

At the top of the breath, close the mouth, relax the chest, and briefly hold the breath by keeping the lips closed. It is not the same to hold the breath by closing the throat or stiffening the chest. Next, allow the lips to open, and let the air fall out of the body through the mouth. As the lips open, the cheeks and lips will relax and puff out a little, creating a soft puffing sound. Do not blow or control the air from the chest, but rather allow the air simply to fall out of the body. At the end of exhalation, just relax until the next breath is taken and the body will relax even more. It is important not

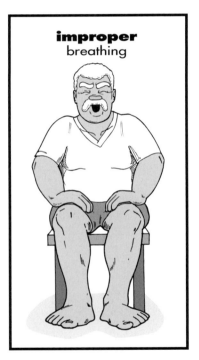

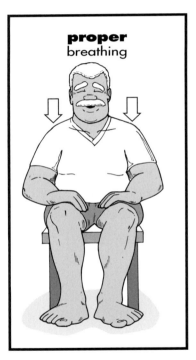

to rush the next breath, but do not wait so long that the body actually *needs* another breath. Concentrate on maintaining a gentle rhythm of approximately six to eight breaths per minute.

It does not matter whether inhalation is through the nose or mouth. Try both, and use the technique that best promotes the level of relaxation necessary for stretch to occur. Many people find that mouth breathing with both inhalation and exhalation works best for them.

The more completely the body and mind can relax, the more the sympathetic nervous system will let the muscles and trigger points soften. As this occurs, the body can be moved in the direction of stretch. Most of the stretching movement will occur during exhalation.

Never Pull or Force the Body to Stretch

The body should be positioned so that it is possible to fully relax the muscles that are about to be stretched. Then, a little tension should be applied to the targeted muscle group following the guidelines of each particular stretch exercise. With the breathing technique described above, focus on relaxing the muscles and allow them to gently lengthen. Continue to gently and slowly move the body in the direction of stretch by taking up the slack that comes from breathing and relaxing.

Do not move any more than just taking up the slack! And just as important, make sure that the movement is very slow and gentle. **Do not move into or try to stretch through a muscle "kink" that will not relax.**

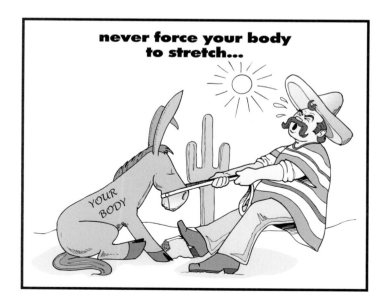

Forcing the stretch in this fashion is likely to cause a flare up of pain from the muscle.

Stop the Stretch

When the muscle stops loosening and there is no more slack, the stretch exercise is **over**. At this time, go on to the next muscle exercise or consider the stretch session to be over. Release the stretch slowly and gently. Following this principle helps **prevent overstretching**.

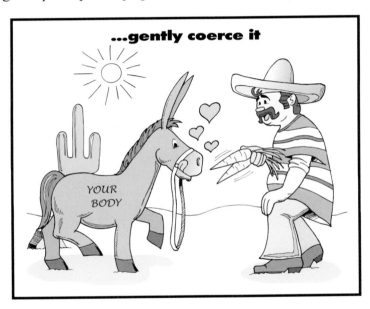

In general, support the body and move to a neutral (non-stretched) position. For side-neck stretches, the hand will move the head back to an upright position and the neck muscles will remain limp (see page 134). Also, the body should center before and after twisting. For lower back quadratus lumborum stretches, stretch forward to center and balance the body before and afterwards (see page 194).

A Bad Example of Stretching

Many people are taught to stretch their pectoralis muscles (the front of the chest) by leaning into a doorway and holding the door frame with the hands as the body leans forwards. In this posture, the pectoralis muscles are keeping the body from falling forward and landing face down on the floor.

It is not possible to stretch a muscle that is contracting to hold up the body!

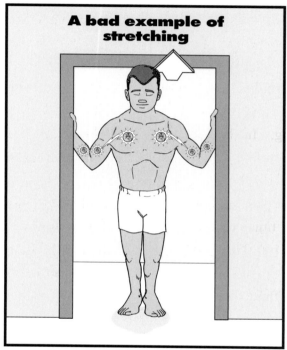

A bad example of stretching

Muscles can only be stretched effectively when they can be made totally limp. A better method of pectoralis stretching is illustrated on page 156.

How Many Times Each Day to Stretch

Imagine a rubber band. Each time it is stretched out, it contracts back to its original shape. The body is very similar to this rubber band and muscles remember being tight. If they are stretched only once or twice each day, the muscles will contract back to their previous level of tightness before the next stretch is performed.

© 1999 blatman / ekvall

Now, imagine what happens to a rubber band when it is stretched out and held out to this length for two to three weeks. In this case, the rubber band never returns to its original and shorter length. It seems to "forget" its previous state of tension.

The body will behave in a similar fashion. If the muscles can be stretched out upon waking, and repeatedly stretched through the day to prevent retightening, the lengthening and relief from pain will become more permanent.

Unlike the rubber band, the body is living tissue. We use our muscles all day and night, and the normal muscle contractions necessary for activity cause tightening. In the absence of stretching, the body progressively tightens. It is therefore imperative that **even the normal and healthy body be stretched once or twice each day.**

Sometimes, people in pain may need to stretch a particular muscle as often as several times each hour. The goal is to prevent the muscle from tightening back up. This is the best guide to answer the question of "how many" times. Each time does not have to take longer than 45 seconds—the time it takes for three or four relaxation breaths.

How far you stretch is not important. The key to improving these pain symptoms, is not allowing the body to tighten back up. Distance will come with time.

Many people feel better for a short while after a massage, chiropractic, or physical therapy session, only to experience a return of their pain within a few hours. Usually this pain returns as the treated muscles tighten back up. When these treatments are supplemented by the techniques taught in this book, they become more effective and progress is quicker.

Tightening is not a Necessary Part of Aging

Older people who are stiff and have difficulty moving do not simply get this way because of advancing age. They mostly get this way because they did not stretch properly and regularly *as* they aged.

Even people who are "behind the eight ball" can perform the techniques in this book to progressively lengthen and stretch their muscles. Gentle and consistent effort will lead to the best chance for success.

The First Stretch of the Day

The first stretch session of the day should be soon after getting up from sleep. This is the most important stretch of the day and it is one of the most difficult times to stretch. The body may be stiff and sore and the person may be sleepy and running late. Do whatever it takes to commit five to ten minutes to using the ball and stretching first thing in the morning.

It is easier to stretch muscles if the ball techniques are performed first. Moist heat also helps muscles to stretch more easily. Make this first and most difficult stretch of the day easier by using the ball and then warming up in the shower first. If

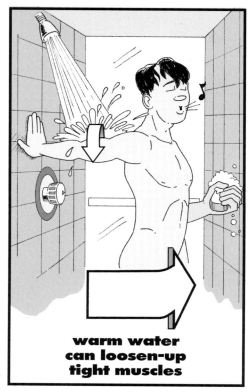

warm water can loosen-up tight muscles

possible, allow the water to spray upon the muscles being stretched. This will be more difficult for muscles of the lower back and buttocks. These should be stretched after warming in the shower. If a chair can be used in the shower area, it is possible to stretch the lower back and buttocks.

If you do not have a chronic pain condition, this first morning "ball and stretch" may be all you need to do for usual body maintenance.

The Second Most Important Stretch of the Day

The second most important stretch of the day is done shortly before going to bed. It is often difficult because by that time of the day many people are just too tired to care. Your recovery will move along faster if you can discipline yourself to stretch before bedtime. Relaxing the muscles before bed will also help relax your mind, allowing for better sleep. In addition, this stretch session will decrease the soreness you typically feel upon arising in the morning and the pain that awakens you at night.

Other Stretches During the Day

For the person actively treating a myofascial pain condition, it may be necessary to stretch a particular muscle every hour or so to keep it from tightening back up. During these subsequent stretch sessions it is not so important for the muscle to be fully stretched as it is important to keep it from tightening back up. This effort does not take very long; a single muscle can be effectively lengthened in only 30–45 seconds, with three or four effective breaths as described above. If time is limited, only stretch the muscle that was tightest during earlier stretches that day, or the muscles identified as a primary cause of the pain pattern being treated.

Stretch Before and After Exercise

The next most important stretching of the day is performed before and after exercise. Everyone knows that athletes stretch before and after their sporting activity. In a similar fashion, we are all athletes. We may not be playing professional or amateur sports, but the principles remain the same. For the less active person, cleaning a room may be the most physically and athletically challenging activity of the day. If there is an activity that typically causes pain to flare, be sure to use the ball and stretch before and after performing that activity. It may also be necessary to take breaks every

stretch

30 minutes for additional ball use and stretching. People who are more fragile should use the ball and stretch before and after even simple activities. Examples include washing dishes, cleaning a room, cooking, and walking.

Does Stretching Before Sports Cause Injury

I have heard a person say that his tennis pro advised him that stretching was not necessary before playing tennis. This person was advised that stretching could cause injury, and that all that was necessary was to warm up using gentle strokes and good body motion for a few minutes before playing. This is utter nonsense. A gentle warmup may be enough only if the person never hits hard or stretches far to reach a ball during play. For most players, this is not realistic.

It is important to stretch before and afterward weightlifting. Many people relish the tight muscular feel to their bodies after weightlifting. This should not be a goal of lifting. Instead, lift for tone and strength, and follow the exercise with stretching so that the body feels loose and comfortable afterwards. The post-lifting stretch also helps prevent post-exercise soreness that is usually noticed 3–24 hours later.

Following the guidelines presented in this section will help to prevent injury from overstretching.

How Does Fibromyalgia Change This Program

People with fibromyalgia have a nervous system that may be more sensitive to pain. Their body may be tighter and less responsive to stretching. Typically, however, they have many myofascial trigger points throughout their musculature that are causing much of their pain pattern. The techniques presented in this book are tried and proven with fibromyalgia patients, as well as athletes. Fibromyalgia patients will need to be patient, working on their bodies more gently and for shorter periods of time. They should also be attentive to their need for drinking water.

If the stretch techniques are causing more pain, you are going too far, too fast. Slow down and be much more gentle. Even if you do not feel anything pulling as you stretch, back off. Your body is still saying that you are going too far, too fast.

stretch

stretching
part 2
STRETCHING POSITIONS

NECK and HEAD

There are several neck muscles that contribute to head and neck pain. These include muscles along the spine from the scalp to the middle back (paraspinal), deep muscles of the back of the neck (suboccipital), muscles of the sides of the neck (scalene and sternocleidomastoid), muscles that lift the shoulder blade towards the base of the skull (levator scapulae), and the surface muscles that span from the base of the skull to the upper shoulders and down to the middle of the back (trapezius).

THREE NECK STRETCHES

These stretches are the basic motions for stretching the muscles listed above. They are important for relieving headache pain, neck pain, upper back pain, and arm pain.

Always use the ball techniques first. It makes the stretches easier to perform.

To perform these stretches, the *hands* are used to guide and move the head and neck. It is not possible to effectively stretch the neck muscles by simply tilting the head to the side. Tilting the head requires muscles on the side of the neck to contract. While muscles on the opposite side of the neck may seem to stretch, they cannot truly lengthen with this motion, and the net effect is that the cervical spine will compress. **To lengthen neck muscles, neck motion must be guided and executed with the hands.**

General Positions

The motions for these stretches can be performed in a seated or standing position. One hand will hold the head and the other hand may anchor the shoulder and upper body.

In a seated position, the shoulder can be anchored by gently grasping underneath the chair. Be sure to keep the shoulder and upper arm relaxed, and in a neutral posture. Do not grasp so low that excess tension is created between the neck and shoulder.

Shoulders and hips must always remain parallel. The anchoring part should be skipped if arm length or chair design contribute to awkward tilting of the body (see diagrams **s-1** and **s-2**).

Without force, gently curl the fingers to hold the edge of the chair and

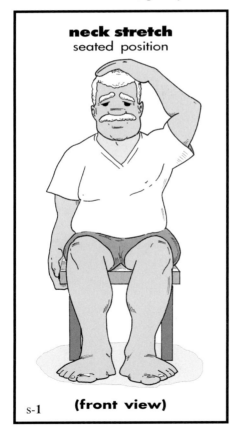

neck stretch
seated position

s-1 **(front view)**

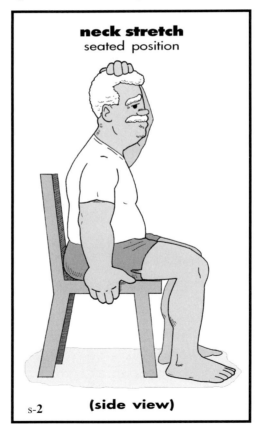

neck stretch
seated position

s-2 **(side view)**

focus on using only the forearm muscles to gently stabilize that side of the body.

In a standing position it may be less convenient to anchor one side. However, in the shower it may be possible to gently hold the wall soap dish as an anchor. Another idea is to use a Theraband™ (rubber tube or strap), with the ends held underneath the feet and one hand gently grasping the loop (see diagram **s-3**).

If these ideas are not practical, gently perform the stretch without anchoring one side. With proper relaxation and technique, the stretch can be just as effective in either a seated or standing position.

Use the free hand to gently hold and guide the head. Place this hand gently on top of the head with the fingertips relaxed against the opposite side of the head, well above the ear.

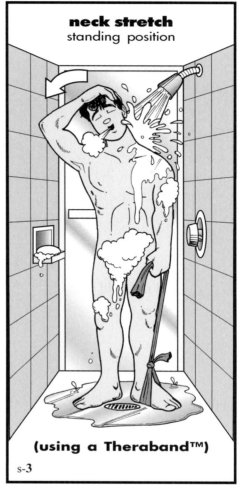

neck stretch
standing position

(using a Theraband™)

s-**3**

Precautions

Always start these stretches with upright posture and no tilt of the head. Also, and most importantly, **do not pull on the head**. The object of this stretch is to relax the muscles of the neck and upper back and **NOT** to get the ear down to touch the shoulder! During stretch recovery, use the hand to guide the head back upright. **Do not** use the neck muscles to straighten the neck and upright the head.

It is usually not a good idea to use the muscle under the arm (upper latissimus) to stabilize and hold the shoulder down. This muscle is already working too hard by opposing the tight upper trapezius muscle. It may be very susceptible to activation of its latent trigger points, and it can cause a major pain pattern (see page 46).

➠POSITION 1

This stretch exercise is started in an upright position with the head facing forward. Place the hand gently on top of the head with the fingers resting on the top and over the side of the head as shown in the picture (see diagrams **s-1** and **s-2**). The elbow should be out to the side, and not held back so far that it is uncomfortable.

Stretch

The stretch is performed as the hand gently guides the head to one side. This will encourage length-ening of scalene and upper trapezius musculature. The hand should lead the head *away* from the anchored side and toward the opposite shoulder (see diagram **s-4**). The shoulders should remain relaxed.

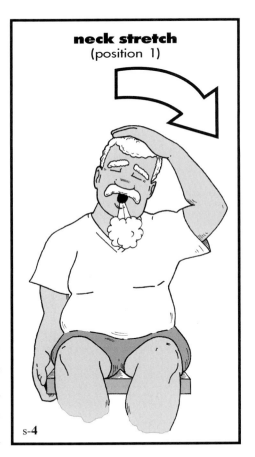

neck stretch
(position 1)

s-4

Relaxation/Breathing

Using relaxation breathing techniques, focus on relaxing both sides of the neck, and move no more than about 15 degrees with each exhalation.

Remember to inhale gently and exhale through the mouth, with a conscious puff of the lips. As the neck muscles relax, guide the head to move sideways just enough to take up the slack of the relaxed muscles. Do not move beyond what will take up the slack. Slower motion and mindful relaxation will result in deeper levels of stretching.

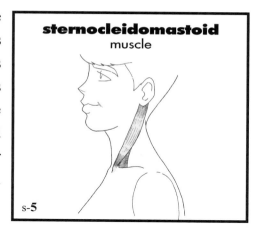

s-5

sternocleidomastoid
muscle

Recovery

After several breaths, there will be no more slack and the muscles will have loosened all they can without being forced. Perhaps take one more breath to be sure, and then gently guide the head back to an upright position with the hand. **Do not use the neck muscles to straighten the neck and upright the head.**

Repeat the exercise on the opposite side. If you are in the shower, turn so that the water sprays the other side.

Helpful Hint

If the side of the neck is stiff and resistant to stretching, acupressure to the **sternocleidomastoid muscle** (see diagram **s-5**) is one technique that may help to release these muscles. The technique is started by firmly grasping the muscle between the thumb and index finger (see diagram **s-6**). Get a good deep grasp of the muscle. Then apply firm pressure

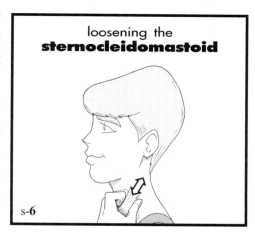

s-6

loosening the
sternocleidomastoid

with a gentle massaging motion to the trigger points in the muscle. It is not unusual to feel the referred pain pattern of the trigger points during this maneuver.

➠POSITION 2

The next stretch exercise starts in an upright position with the head rotated approximately 60° to the side. Place the hand gently on top of the head with the fingers resting on the top and back of the head as shown in the picture (see diagram **s-7**). The elbow should be right in front of the nose with the forearm aligned in the same direction as the head.

The first stretch of the day is best done in the warm shower with the water beating upon the muscles being stretched.

Stretch

This stretch is performed as the hand slowly guides the chin down towards the chest with the nose aimed toward the elbow. This will encourage lengthening of trapezius, posterior cervical, and levator scapulae musculature.

Relaxation/Breathing

Using relaxation breathing techniques, focus on relaxing the entire neck and move no more than about 15 degrees with each exhalation. Remember to inhale gently and exhale through the

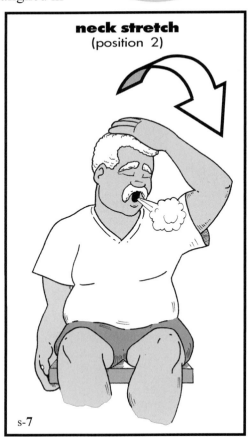

neck stretch
(position 2)

s-7

stretch

139

mouth, with a conscious puff of the lips. Use the hand to gently guide the head downward toward the chest. As the neck muscles relax, guide the head to move just enough to take up the slack of the relaxed muscles. Do not move beyond what will take up the slack. Slower motion and mindful relaxation will result in deeper levels of stretching.

Recovery

After several breaths, there will be no more slack and the muscles will have loosened all they can without being forced. Perhaps take one more breath to be sure, and then gently guide the head back to an upright position with the hand. **Do not use the neck muscles to straighten the neck and upright the head.**

Repeat the exercise on the opposite side. If you are in the shower, turn so that the water sprays the other side.

⇒POSITION 3

This stretch exercise is started in an upright position with the head facing forward. Place the hand gently on top of the head with the fingers resting near the middle and toward the back of the head as shown in the picture (see diagram **s-8**). The elbow should be mostly forward, and the arm and shoulder should not be uncomfortable.

Stretch

The stretch is performed as the hand gently guides the head forward. This will encourage lengthening of the paraspinal muscles in the neck and the paraspinal muscles down to the lower back. The hand should lead the head forward, trying to first tuck the chin. The shoulders should remain relaxed.

Relaxation/Breathing

Using relaxation breathing techniques, focus on relaxing both sides of the neck and move no more than about 15 degrees (or 1 inch) with each exhalation. Remember to inhale gently and exhale through the mouth, with a conscious puff of the lips. As the neck muscles relax, guide the head to move sideways just enough to take up the slack of the relaxed muscles. Do not move beyond what will take up the slack. Slower motion and mindful relaxation will result in deeper levels of stretching.

Recovery

After several breaths, there will be no more slack and the muscles will have loosened all they can without being forced. Perhaps take one more breath to be sure, and then gently guide the head back to an upright position with the hand. **Do not use the neck muscles to straighten the neck and upright the head.**

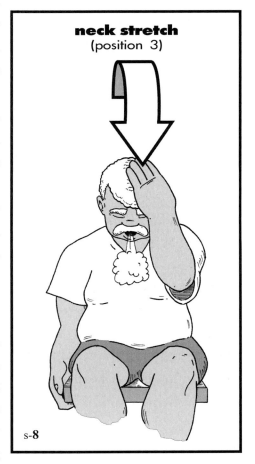

neck stretch
(position 3)

s-**8**

MASSETER AND TEMPORALIS

The masseter muscle works primarily to close the jaw. It gets injured with direct trauma, grinding the teeth, opening the mouth too wide, an unbalanced bite, and chewing gum.

⫸POSITION 1

These muscles can be stretched while sitting, standing, or lying on the back. Start by placing the fingertips of both hands on the sides of the face in front of the middle of the ears (see diagrams **s-9A&B**). Then push in with a level of force that is gentle and firm. This position stretches mostly the masseter muscles.

Precautions

When pushing in against the sides of the face, do not push too hard. This stretch will be helpful even with the gentlest pressure. Be conscious of tension in the back of the neck, and keep this area as relaxed as possible. When doing this stretch in the position of lying on the back, do not apply enough force to lift the head against gravity.

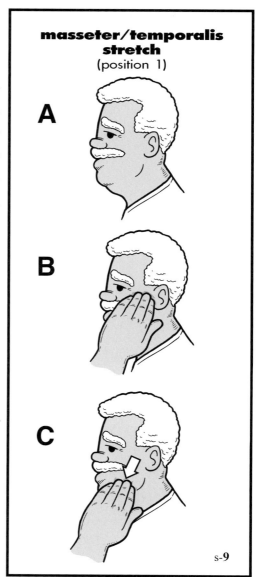

masseter/temporalis stretch
(position 1)

A

B

C

s-9

Stretch

The stretch occurs as the hands are slowly moved towards the feet, with the fingertips dragging the skin and muscles of the sides of the face (see diagram **s-9C**). Keep the finger pressure firm and allow the jaw to open as the stretch proceeds. It should take at least 10–15 seconds to do this stretch.

Relaxation/Breathing

Using relaxation breathing techniques, focus on relaxing the entire jaw. Remember to inhale gently and exhale through the mouth. A conscious puff of the lips may not be possible. Keep the upper back, head, and neck upright. As the jaw muscles relax, allow the jaw to open slowly. The jaw should not be actively opened, and may only move a little bit. Do not move the hands faster than what will take up the slack in the relaxing muscles. Slower motion and mindful relaxation will result in deeper levels of stretching.

Recovery

To recover from this stretch, simply let go and allow the arms to drop to a relaxed position and the mouth to close.

⫸POSITION 2

This stretch should be done lying on the back. The hands should also be washed or gloved. Start by placing the long, index, or both fingers of each hand into the mouth. Then set the fingertips against the bite surface of the bottom teeth in the very back of the mouth (see diagram **s-10**).

Precautions

When pushing down on the teeth, do not apply any force to the lower front teeth. Pushing on the front teeth will tend to compress the jaw joint. The goal of this stretch is to decompress the joint and relax the jaw-closing muscles. Also, take care to apply all the force in a direction directly towards the feet. Do not push the jaw in or pull it out. Lastly, do not push/pull too hard. This stretch will be helpful even with the gentlest pressure. Be conscious of tension in the back of the neck, and keep this area as relaxed as possible. The reason to perform this stretch while lying down is to be more able to gauge the force applied to the teeth, and not apply enough force to lift the head against gravity.

stretch

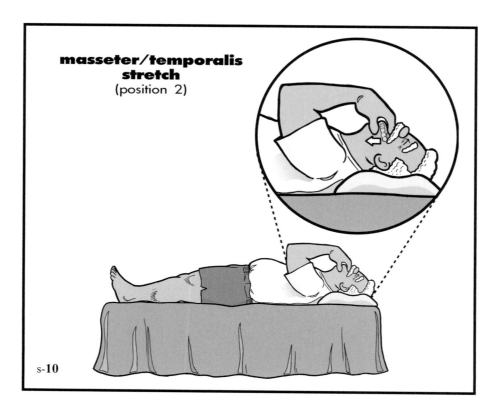

masseter/temporalis
stretch
(position 2)

s-10

Stretch

The stretch occurs as the fingertips gently and firmly push/pull the jaw open (see diagram **s-10**). Visualize lowering the entire jaw assembly and opening the joint. Keep the finger pressure firm and allow the jaw to open as the stretch proceeds.

Relaxation/Breathing

Using relaxation breathing techniques, focus on relaxing the entire jaw and neck. Remember to inhale gently and exhale through the mouth. A conscious puff of the lips will not be possible. Keep the upper back, head, and neck straight and relaxed. As the jaw muscles relax, the jaw will open slowly. Do not actively open the jaw. Also, do not move beyond what will take up the slack in the relaxing muscles. Slower motion and mindful relaxation will result in deeper levels of stretching.

Recovery

To recover from this stretch, simply let go and allow the arms to drop to a relaxed position and the mouth to close.

UPPER BACK, SHOULDER, and CHEST

There are several muscles that contribute to upper back, shoulder, and chest pain. These include muscles over the shoulder blade (infraspinatus), muscles under the arm (upper latissimus, teres major, and teres minor), muscles of the upper chest (pectoralis), muscles under the shoulder blade (subscapularis), and muscles that cover the shoulder joint (deltoid). Some of these muscles (infraspinatus and latissimus) also contribute to arm and hand pain. Muscles covering the shoulder blade (subscapularis and infraspinatus) also contribute to shoulder pain and neck pain (infraspinatus).

INFRASPINATUS

This muscle has the action of rotating the arm outwards. To stretch the muscle, the arm has to be rotated inwards. It is this muscle that gets stretched when children play "elevator" with each other. (This stretch is also used for teres minor trigger points, not separately discussed.)

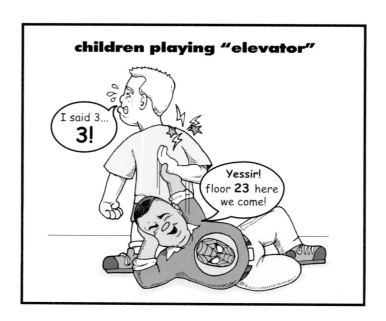

children playing "elevator"

I said 3... **3!**

Yessir! floor **23** here we come!

➠POSITION 1

To start this stretch, first move the forearm and hand behind the back at waist level. Rest the wrist and hand on the top of the buttocks. Reach across the front of the body with the other hand and gently wrap the fingers around the elbow or upper arm (see diagram **s-11**). This position should not be uncomfortable. Some people with shorter arms or tighter muscles may not be able to reach and hold their arm in this fashion, and may be able to hold a shirt sleeve instead.

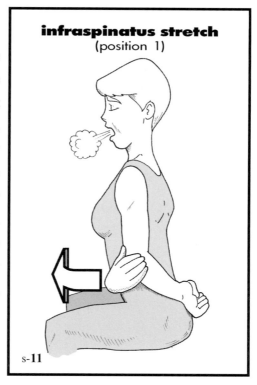

infraspinatus stretch
(position 1)

s-11

Precautions

Do not apply more pressure than just the weight of the arm. Very little motion is needed to stretch this muscle.

Stretch

This stretch is performed by holding the arm and applying gentle pressure. The shoulder will rotate inward and forward just a little. As this happens, the elbow will move toward the front of the body. Very little motion is needed to perform this stretch effectively.

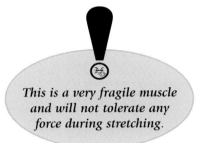

This is a very fragile muscle and will not tolerate any force during stretching.

Relaxation/Breathing

Using relaxation breathing techniques, focus on relaxing the back of the neck, upper back, and shoulder. Remember to inhale gently and exhale through the mouth, with a conscious puff of the lips. The arm and shoulder will move slightly forward guided by the other hand. Slower motion and mindful relaxation will result in deeper levels of stretching.

Recovery

To recover from this stretch, let go of the arm, and let the hand behind the back fall to the side.

Repeat the exercise on the

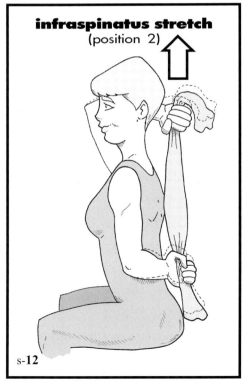

infraspinatus stretch
(position 2)

s-12

opposite side.

➠POSITION 2

Hold a towel with one end in each hand as shown in the picture (see diagram **s-12**).

Precautions

Keep the shoulder and arm being stretched as relaxed as possible. A little motion means a lot of stretch. Do not try to move too far during a single stretch session, and do not stretch into pain.

Stretch

The stretch occurs as the upper arm is raised, causing the lower arm to move upwards toward the middle back (see diagram **s-12**).

Relaxation/Breathing

Using relaxation breathing techniques, focus on relaxing the back of the neck, upper back, and shoulder. Remember to inhale gently and exhale through the mouth, with a conscious puff of the lips. Use the upper hand to slowly pull the towel upward, thereby raising the lower hand and internally rotating the shoulder. Slower motion and mindful relaxation will result in deeper levels of stretching.

Recovery

Slowly lower the upper arm and let the lower arm fall. Then release the grasp of the lower arm on the towel and let the arm fall to the side. Repeat the exercise on the opposite side.

➠POSITION 3

Place both hands behind the back and hold one with the other. If the arms are short, simply interlock a few fingers. Bend forward at the waist,

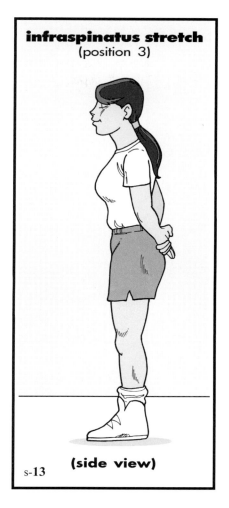

infraspinatus stretch
(position 3)

(side view)

s-13

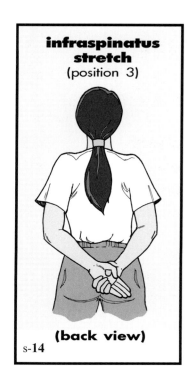

infraspinatus stretch
(position 3)

(back view)

s-14

allowing the elbows to fall forward. Also allow the neck to relax and the head to hang down (see diagrams **s-13 and s-14**).

Precautions

Allow the force of gravity alone to make this stretch happen. Do not use the muscles of the front of the chest to force more motion. Try to leave the neck as limp as possible, letting the head hang from the shoulders. Keeping the head up may cause tightening of paraspinal muscles from the head to the tailbone.

149

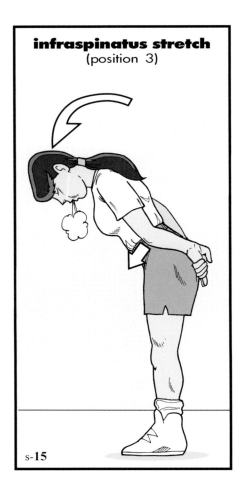

infraspinatus stretch
(position 3)

s-15

Stretch

The stretch occurs as the elbows fall toward the floor (see diagram **s-15**). In this position, both sides of the body will be stretched at the same time.

Relaxation/Breathing

Using relaxation breathing techniques, focus on relaxing the upper back, neck, and shoulders. Allow gravity to pull the elbows forward and down toward the floor. With additional breaths, the elbows should move further. Slower motion and mindful relaxation will result in deeper levels of stretching.

Recovery

Slowly stand upright, let go of the hands, and allow the arms to fall to the sides of the body.

SUBSCAPULARIS

This shoulder muscle has the action of rotating the arm inwards. To stretch this muscle, the arm has to be rotated outwards. This muscle gets injured with side-arm and over-arm throwing, forehand racket sports, and carrying or pushing objects in front of the body between both hands. (This stretch is also used for teres major trigger points, not separately discussed.)

⇒POSITION

This stretch is easily performed standing next to a door frame, with the frame about a forearm's length away from the side of the body. With the arm of the shoulder being stretched hanging by the side, bend the elbow 90° and gently grip the moulding at the side of the door frame. Place the other hand on this arm close to the elbow, and just stabilize the arm, keeping the elbow by the waist (see diagram **s-16**).

Precautions

This muscle is not very strong compared to the muscles of the arm. It also does not need much motion in order to stretch. **This**

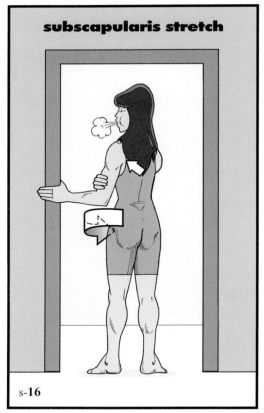

subscapularis stretch

s-**16**

exercise must be done very slowly and very gently. Do not push to stretch further.

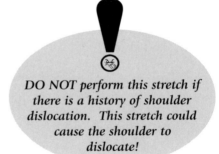

Stretch

The stretch occurs as the body is rotated away from the door frame. In many people, the body will rotate until the forearm is straight out to the side. People who are more flexible will be able to rotate farther, so that the forearm is directed more backwards (see diagram **s-16**).

Relaxation/Breathing

Using relaxation breathing techniques, focus on relaxing the shoulder and arm. Remember to inhale gently and exhale through the mouth, with a conscious puff of the lips. Slowly rotate the body away from the door frame. Slower motion and mindful relaxation will result in deeper levels of stretching.

Recovery

To recover from stretching in this position, rotate the body toward the door frame and let go, allowing the forearm to drop to the side. Repeat the exercise with the opposite arm.

UPPER LATISSIMUS

The latissimus muscle goes from the shoulder blade to the pelvic bone at the waist. Its action is to pull the arm downwards toward the waist. To stretch the upper part of this muscle, the arm has to be raised overhead and then the shoulder blade needs to be elevated. The technique for stretching the lower part of this muscle is described on pages 196–200. This muscle gets injured by doing pull ups, computer mouse work, holding the steering wheel tightly, and carrying objects against the side of the body.

⤳POSITION 1

From a standing position, reach up with one arm at a time and gently hold onto something that is at a comfortable height overhead. A chin-up bar is most effective. Use only enough grip strength to hold on to the bar, leaving the arm and shoulder as limp as possible (see diagram **s-17**).

Precautions

This is an easy muscle to overstretch and special care should be taken to be gentle. **Do not hang from the hand**. Most of the body's weight should be held with the legs.

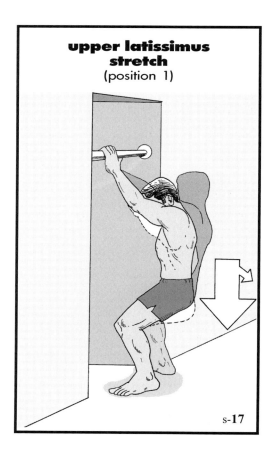

upper latissimus
stretch
(position 1)

s-**17**

Stretch

The stretch occurs as the knees are allowed to bend, letting the body sink downwards (see diagram **s-17**).

Relaxation/Breathing

Using relaxation breathing techniques, focus on relaxing the under arm, shoulder, and neck. With additional breaths, slowly bend the knees and allow the shoulder to be elevated so the "hip-shoulder" length increases.

Recovery

To recover from this stretch, simply straighten the knees and stand up. Repeat the exercise with the opposite arm.

⟶POSITION 2

Bend forward at the waist and hold onto an object at approximately waist level, such as a door knob. Position the feet a little in front of the waist so that the lower body is leaning backwards. Use only enough grip strength to hold on to the door knob, leaving the arm and shoulder as limp as possible (see diagram **s-18**).

Precautions

This is an easy muscle to overstretch and special care should be taken to be gentle. Do not pull and do not apply force from the legs. When recovering from this stretch, do not pull the body up with the arm holding the door knob.

Stretch

The stretch occurs as the lower body leans backwards, with the door knob applying a gentle force to raise the shoulder towards the head (see diagram **s-18**).

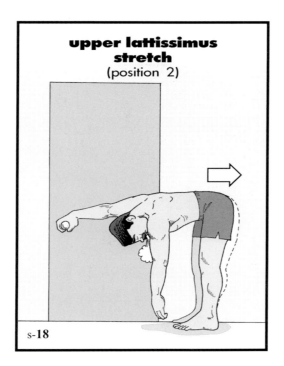

upper lattissimus stretch
(position 2)

s-18

Relaxation/Breathing

Using relaxation breathing techniques, focus on relaxing the entire side of the body, including the shoulder and arm. Remember to inhale gently and exhale through the mouth, with a conscious puff of the lips. With additional breaths, slowly allow the shoulder to be elevated so the "hip-shoulder" length increases. Slower motion and mindful relaxation will result in deeper levels of stretching.

Repeat this exercise on the opposite side.

Recovery

To recover from this stretch, bend the knee closest to the door, lift the opposite foot off the floor and move it forwards. Push off the back foot and take small steps forward, using the door knob to assist in standing up.

Repeat the exercise on the opposite side.

PECTORALIS

The pectoralis muscles pull the arms forward across the chest, and also pull the shoulders forward. If these muscles are tight, they keep the shoulders forward and this causes an increase in tension for the muscles of the upper back. For the upper back to stay loose, the front of the chest must be stretched. To stretch this muscle, the arms have to be held out to the side, and then moved back behind the body. This muscle gets injured with pushing forward and away from the body, holding an object between the hands in front of the body, and raking.

Do not lean forward and do not contract the pectoralis muscles during this stretch.

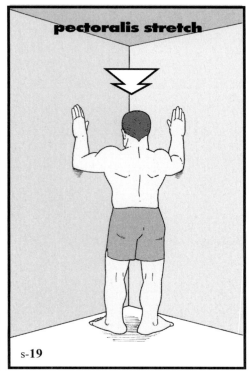

pectoralis stretch

s-19

⟶POSITION

Hold both arms up like a robber just came up behind you and said "*stick em up.*" Walk into the corner and place both hands and forearms against the walls. Keep the body as upright as possible (see diagram **s-19**).

Precautions

Do not lean forward. This might cause the pectoralis muscles to tighten in order to protect the face from hitting the wall.

Stretch

Keep the body balanced on the feet and slowly walk forward, moving the nose into the corner. As this happens, the front of the chest will be stretched (see diagram **s-19**).

Relaxation/Breathing

Using relaxation breathing techniques, focus on relaxing the neck, shoulder, and chest. Remember to inhale gently and exhale through the mouth, with a conscious puff of the lips. Slowly take small steps toward the corner, allowing the chest and front of the shoulders to separate. Slower motion and mindful relaxation will result in deeper levels of stretching.

Recovery

To recover from stretching in this position, take small steps backwards, and then let the arms fall to the sides of the body.

DELTOID

The deltoid muscle moves the arm at the shoulder, in forward, sideways, and backward directions. There are three parts to this muscle, and the front and back parts are stretched separately. There is no optimal way to stretch the middle part because the chest is directly in the way. The deltoid muscle gets injured with repetitive lifting above chest height, bruising, and use as a site for medical injections.

⫸POSITION 1
ANTERIOR (FRONT) PART OF THE DELTOID

To stretch the front part of the muscle, the arm must be moved behind and across the back of the body. Start by putting the arm behind the back,

157

and then grasp the elbow with the other hand (see diagram **s-20**). If there is not enough flexibility to begin in this position, then grasp the wrist with the other hand (see diagram **s-21**).

Precautions

During this stretch, and during positioning prior to the stretch, it is very important to keep all of the shoulder musculature as relaxed and limp as possible. Some people performing this stretch may tend to work too hard to put the arm behind their back, activating trigger points in the upper back and shoulder (upper latissimus, rhomboid, and subscapularis) in the process.

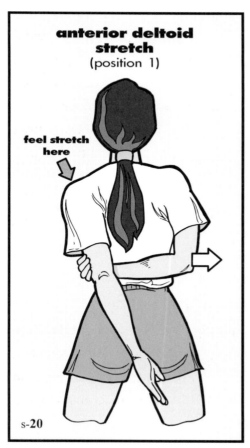

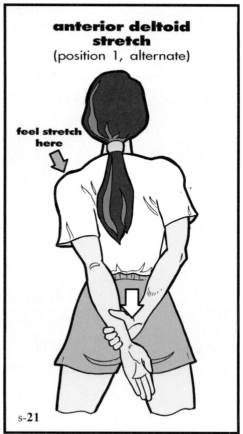

Stretch

The stretch occurs as the arm is pulled further across the back of the body by the opposite arm (see diagrams **s-20** and **s-21**). Leave the fingers of the grasping hand relatively loose and gently pull so that there is tension on the shoulder being stretched. Then gently curl the grasping fingers to pull the arm a little further across the back of the body. When flexibility is not great enough and the wrist is being grasped, the stretching force will be gentler because there is less mechanical advantage. The best effort will be to pull the wrist gently down towards the feet.

Relaxation/Breathing

Using relaxation breathing techniques, focus on relaxing the entire shoulder. Remember to inhale gently and exhale through the mouth, with a conscious puff of the lips. Keep the upper back, head, and neck upright. As the shoulder muscles relax, curl the fingers a little more, applying more force to the elbow area and pulling the arm a little further across the back. Do not move beyond what will take up the slack in the relaxing muscles. Slower motion and mindful relaxation will result in deeper levels of stretching.

Recovery

To recover from this stretch, simply let go and allow the arms to drop to a relaxed position.

⟾POSITION 2
POSTERIOR (BACK) PART OF THE DELTOID

To stretch the back part of the muscle, the arm must be moved forward and across the front of the body. Start by putting the arm across the chest, and then grasp the elbow or just above the elbow with the other hand (see diagram **s-22**). If there is not enough flexibility to begin in this position, then grasp the forearm near the elbow.

stretch

Precautions

During this stretch, and during positioning prior to the stretch, it is very important to keep all of the shoulder musculature as relaxed and limp as possible. Some people performing this stretch may tend to pull the arm across their body by using the chest muscles, activating trigger points in the pectoralis muscles. Also, pulling on the arm to do the stretch may activate trigger points in the biceps, or in the upper back and shoulder (rhomboid, middle trapezius, deltoid) muscles of the other arm.

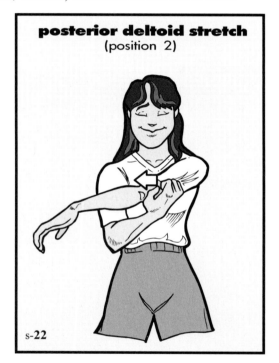

posterior deltoid stretch
(position 2)

s-22

Stretch

The stretch occurs as the arm is pulled further across the front of the body by the opposite arm (see diagram **s-22**).

Relaxation/Breathing

Using relaxation breathing techniques, focus on relaxing the entire shoulder. Remember to inhale gently and exhale through the mouth, with a conscious puff of the lips. Keep the upper back, head, and neck upright. As the shoulder muscles relax, continue to apply gentle pressure to the elbow area, pulling the arm a little further across the chest. Do not move beyond what will take up the slack in the relaxing muscles. Slower motion and mindful relaxation will result in deeper levels of stretching.

Recovery

To recover from this stretch, simply let go and allow the arms to drop to a relaxed position.

⟶POSITION 3
POSTERIOR (BACK) PART OF THE DELTOID

This part of the muscle can also be stretched in a lying down position. People who have limited upper back strength or chronic upper back and shoulder pain may find this stretch position to be best. Start by lying on the side with the arm to be stretched placed straight out in front and slightly down towards the waist (see diagram **s-23**).

Precautions

During this stretch do not turn too far or too quickly. A little bit of rotation translates to a lot of stretch. Make sure that the other hand and arm control all the motion of rotation during the stretch. The shoulder muscles being stretched must remain limp. Also it is very important to keep the neck as relaxed as possible.

Stretch

The stretch occurs as the body is rolled toward lying on the stomach (see diagram **s-24**). Support the body with the other hand (left hand in diagram **s-24**), and only drop the hand over the edge of the bed if there is enough flexibility.

stretch

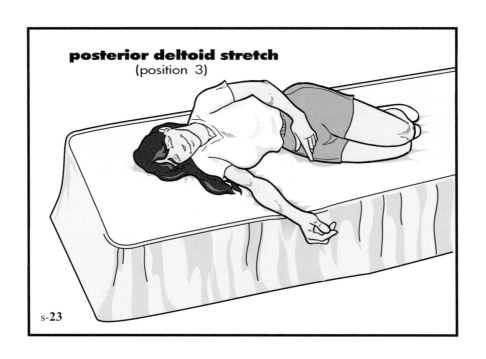

posterior deltoid stretch
(position 3)

s-23

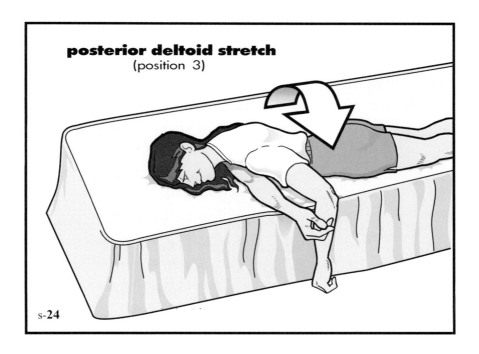

posterior deltoid stretch
(position 3)

s-24

Relaxation/Breathing

Using relaxation breathing techniques, focus on relaxing the entire shoulder. Remember to inhale gently and exhale through the mouth, with a conscious puff of the lips. Keep the upper back, head, and neck in a good upright posture, even while lying down. As the shoulder muscles relax, continue too apply gentle pressure by turning more and forcing the arm a little closer to the chest. Do not move beyond what will take up the slack in the relaxing muscles. Slower motion and mindful relaxation will result in deeper levels of stretching.

Recovery

To recover from this stretch, simply push with the other hand and rotate the body back onto the side or back.

UPPER EXTREMITIES

There are several muscles that contribute to arm and hand pain. These include muscles along the front of the arm (biceps), muscles along the back of the arm (triceps), muscles of the top of the forearm (wrist dorsiflexors and finger extensors), muscles of the underside of the forearm (wrist palmar flexors and finger flexors), muscles of the thumb (thenar), and muscles of the hand (lumbricales). Infraspinatus and upper latissimus muscles can also cause arm, forearm, and hand pain. These muscles are discussed in the upper back and chest section (see pages 145 and 152).

Tension in some of these muscles (biceps, wrist palmar flexor, and thenar) contributes to carpal tunnel syndrome. Stretching these muscles can help relieve carpal tunnel syndrome.

Tension in other muscles (wrist dorsiflexor) contributes to tennis elbow. Stretching these muscles can help relieve tennis elbow.

Tension in hand muscles (lumbricales) contributes to hand and finger pain. Stretching these muscles can relieve hand pain.

CARPAL TUNNEL SYNDROME (CTS)

The carpal tunnel is a canal through the wrist that is bordered on the top by the wrist bones and on the bottom (palm side) by a thick ligament called

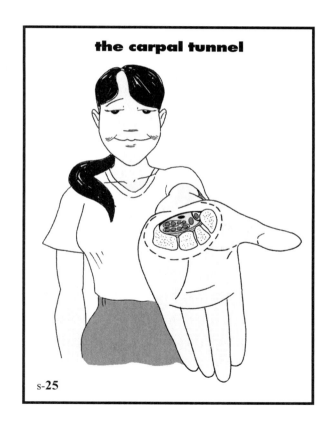

the carpal tunnel

s-25

the transverse carpal ligament. Tendons and a nerve pass through the carpal tunnel. The tendons curl the fingers to make a fist, and the "median" nerve enables us to feel our thumb, index, long, and half of the ring finger. The other half of the ring finger and the pinkie finger are supplied by the "ulnar" nerve which does not go through the carpal tunnel (see diagram **s-25**).

WHAT CAUSES CARPAL TUNNEL SYNDROME?

Old Theory

Carpal tunnel syndrome (CTS) has traditionally been thought of as an inflammatory condition caused by repetitive strain of the forearm, wrist and hand. Repetitive use of the fingers and bending of the wrist is thought to cause tendons in the wrist to become inflamed and swollen. Unfortunately, there is no extra room in the canal to accommodate this swelling, and when the median nerve gets pinched, the fingers (all but the pinkie) may get numb and the wrist and forearm may become painful. Bending the wrist in most any direction causes the canal size to shrink, also aggravating or causing symptoms.

Traditional Treatment

First line treatment includes wearing a brace so that the wrist doesn't bend as much, especially at night. This can be very helpful, particularly for people who sleep with their wrist(s) bent. Wearing the brace during the work day can also be helpful, but some people try to use their hands too much and "fight" the brace. These people sometimes find that wearing the brace aggravates their condition.

The tendon inflammation is traditionally treated with prescription anti-inflammatory medication. Sometimes cortisone, a stronger anti-inflammatory medication, is injected into the carpal tunnel to decrease this inflammation.

When these treatments are not effective, an operation may be performed to cut the transverse carpal ligament, increasing the size of the canal. Surgery often relieves the symptoms, but when people return to work (or whatever activity that contributed most to the problem), the condition often recurs.

New Theory

Fortunately, there is a new way to think about carpal tunnel syndrome. Recent research has demonstrated that the theorized inflammation of the wrist tendons does not occur. In addition, we have found that specific exercises can be effective for treating and preventing carpal tunnel syndrome.

The cause of carpal tunnel syndrome can actually start with the biceps muscle of the arm. People who use their wrists and fingers a lot generally support and stabilize their forearms and hands with a sustained contraction of the biceps muscle. This continuous contraction of the biceps muscle eventually leads to tightening of the connective tissue called fascia, that runs through the muscle and the front of the arm. The biceps muscle crosses the elbow, and as the arm fascia tightens, so does the fascia of the forearm. With time, this tightening extends to the fascia of the wrist and the transverse carpal ligament. As this occurs, the carpal tunnel gets smaller! In other words, *CTS is not usually caused by tendon inflammation and swelling, but rather by fascial tightening and shrinking carpal canal size. This shrinking of the canal compresses the median nerve and the flexor tendons.*

New Treatment

The exercises described here are designed to assist in the treatment and prevention of carpal tunnel syndrome. Positions and motions described here are designed to stretch the musculature and fascia of the arm, forearm, wrist, and hand. Stretches for each of these body areas are discussed separately.

166

Some of these areas can be stretched with more than one technique. Each person is encouraged to try all of the techniques, and then focus efforts more on those that are most helpful and effective. Every stretch does not need to be performed during each session. The ones that work best should be performed several times each day, starting soon after awakening. Stretches for the tightest or most overworked muscles may need to be performed up to 15 times each day. As activities during the day cause muscles and fascia to tighten, stretching must be repeated to ensure that the tightening does not progress.

In addition to solo stretches, there is instruction for a two person stretch to lengthen the transverse carpal ligament (see pages 179–181) This is the ligament that is cut during carpal tunnel surgery. Stretching it is generally very helpful.

BICEPS

The biceps muscle bends the elbow, assists in bringing the arm forward at the shoulder and rotates the forearm outwards (thumb up and away from the body). To stretch this muscle, the elbow needs to be straightened. Deeper stretch occurs when the upper arm is moved upwards and out to the side of the body. This stretch position also stretches the fascia of the front of the arm. The biceps muscle gets injured with lifting, holding or carrying objects, climbing (a rope or ladder), and using a screw driver.

➡️POSITION 1

In order to stretch this muscle, the elbow is held straight and the shoulder joint is moved into extension, positioning the arm behind the body. The arm being stretched is positioned directly behind and almost even with the shoulder joint (see diagram **s-26**). If the arm is too tight to begin in this position then start it at a lower, more comfortable height. The hand is placed

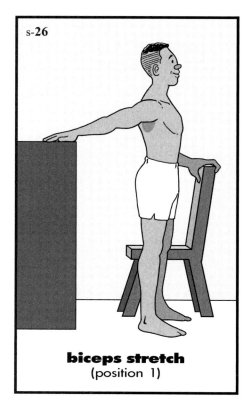

biceps stretch
(position 1)

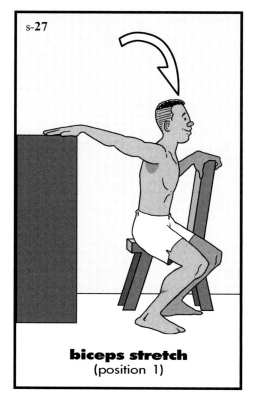

biceps stretch
(position 1)

with the palm downwards and resting on a counter or shelf. The shoulder musculature should be totally limp. The elbow is held in a straight position by the stretch, and the arm and forearm musculature is also totally limp.

Precautions

During this stretch, and during positioning prior to the stretch, it is very important to keep all of the shoulder musculature relaxed and limp. People performing this stretch tend to actively extend the shoulder (moving the arm behind and lifting it up). This is likely to activate painful trigger points in upper back and shoulder (trapezius, rhomboid, and subscapularis) musculature. With stretch recovery, do not try to lift the arm up and around the body using the posterior shoulder muscles.

Stretch

The stretch occurs as the shoulder joint is moved further into extension (arm behind the body). To accomplish this leave the shoulder musculature limp and allow the countertop to stabilize the hand and forearm, while lowering the body toward the ground by bending the knees (see diagram **s-27**).

Relaxation/Breathing

Using relaxation breathing techniques, focus on relaxing the upper back, shoulder, and arm. Remember to inhale gently and exhale through the mouth, with a conscious puff of the lips. A pulling sensation and perhaps some burning will be felt along the biceps, and possibly up into the shoulder and down into the hand. As the shoulder and arm muscles relax, continue to bend the knees further and lower the body just enough to take up the slack of the relaxing

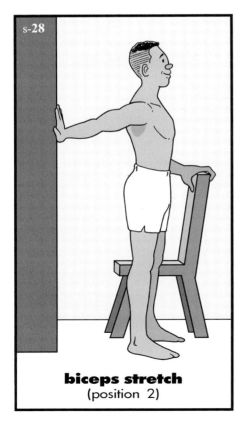

biceps stretch
(position 2)

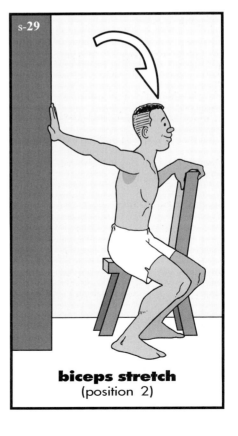

biceps stretch
(position 2)

muscles. Do not move beyond what will take up the slack. Slower motion and mindful relaxation will result in deeper levels of stretching.

Recovery

When the biceps muscle has released, stand up and allow the arm to fall gently to the side of the body. Do not try to lift the arm up and around the body using the posterior shoulder muscles.

Repeat the exercise on the other side.

⫸POSITION 2

Alternatively, the biceps can be stretched in another standing position. Reach the arm behind and almost at shoulder level with the hand (fingers up) pressed into the wall. Relax the shoulder and support the hand with pressure against the wall (see diagram **s-28**). The stretch occurs as the knees are bent and the body is lowered (see diagram **s-29**). Relaxation breathing and stretching is the same as for Position 1 described in biceps stretch above (see page 167).

TRICEPS

The triceps muscle straightens the elbow and assists in moving the arm backwards behind the body. To stretch this muscle, the elbow must be bent. Deeper stretch occurs when the upper arm is moved to a position straight up and next to the head. This stretch position also stretches the fascia of the back of the arm and side of the body. The triceps muscle gets injured with punching, pushing objects, and doing push-ups. Although this muscle is not directly involved in causing carpal tunnel syndrome, it should be stretched once or twice per day if the biceps are really tight. In addition, this muscle acts over two joints. To stretch it effectively, both the shoulder and elbow joints must be positioned.

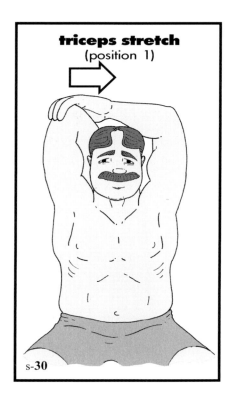

triceps stretch
(position 1)

s-**30**

⫸POSITION 1

Position the shoulder with the arm straight overhead and then bend the elbow, allowing the hand to drop behind the head. Hold the upward arm near the elbow with the other hand, and place the thumb on the forearm to push and bend the elbow further. The hand will fall toward the area of the spine between the shoulder blades (see diagram **s-30**).

Precautions

The arm being stretched should remain limp and relaxed. Do not contract the biceps to stretch the triceps.

Stretch

The hand holding the elbow lifts upward on the arm and at the same time the thumb pushes on the forearm to bend the elbow a little more (see diagram

s-30). A pulling sensation may be felt along the arm in the area of the triceps muscle. Additionally, pulling may be felt along the side of the body.

Relaxation/Breathing

Using relaxation breathing techniques, focus on relaxing the neck, shoulder, under arm, and upper back. Remember to inhale gently and exhale through the mouth, with a conscious puff of the lips. With additional breaths, think of pulling up with the hand to lift the elbow higher, and apply more force with the thumb to bend the elbow. Slower motion and mindful relaxation

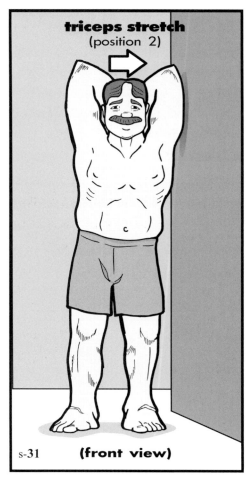

triceps stretch
(position 2)

s-31   **(front view)**

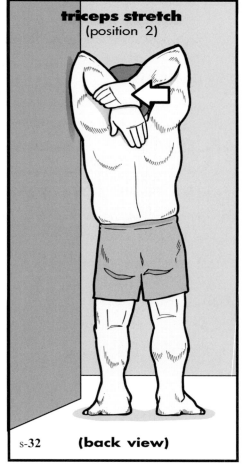

triceps stretch
(position 2)

s-32   **(back view)**

will result in deeper levels of stretching.

Recovery

To recover from this stretch, slowly release the elbow, allowing the arm to drop to the side of the body.

Repeat this exercise on the opposite side.

⟶POSITION 2

This position is likely to be best for the person who has pain from trigger points in upper shoulder and neck muscles. Use a wall to position the shoulder with the arm up overhead and then bend the elbow, allowing the hand to drop behind the head. Hold the upward arm near the wrist with the other hand (see diagrams **s-31 and s-32**).

Precautions

The arm being stretched should remain limp and relaxed. Do not contract the biceps to stretch the triceps.

Stretch

The hand holding the wrist pushes toward the wall, bending the elbow (see diagram **s-32**). A pulling sensation may be felt along the arm in the area of the triceps muscle. Additionally, pulling may be felt along the side of the body.

Relaxation/Breathing

Using relaxation breathing techniques, focus on relaxing the neck, shoulder, under arm, and upper back. Remember to inhale gently and exhale through the mouth, with a conscious puff of the lips. With additional breaths, push on the wrist and bend the elbow further. Slower motion and mindful relaxation will result in deeper levels of stretching.

Recovery

To recover from this stretch, slowly move away from the wall, allowing the arm to drop to the side of the body.

Repeat this exercise on the opposite side.

FOREARM (CARPAL TUNNEL SYNDROME, GOLFER'S ELBOW)

There are several muscles on the palm side of the forearm that contribute to carpal tunnel syndrome (CTS) and golfer's elbow. These include the wrist flexors (flexor carpi ulnaris and radialis) and finger flexors (flexor digitorum group). Trigger points in these muscles may also contribute to pain in the forearm, wrist, and hand. Contraction of these muscles flexes the wrist and curls the fingers. Repetitive use of these muscles is associated with CTS. Frequent breaks and stretching through the day can improve symptoms related to these muscles. To stretch these muscles, the fingers and elbow are held straight and the wrist is bent backwards with the other hand.

⇒POSITION

This stretch can be performed in a standing or sitting position. The forearm being stretched is positioned near the middle of the body, extending downwards and in front of the body with the palm upwards. The shoulder, neck, and upper arm should remain relaxed. The fingers of the hand to be stretched are held so that the fingers of the other hand contact the palm side, and the thumb of the other hand presses into the top side (dorsum) of the fingers to keep the finger joints (IP joints) straight. The index finger forms a bar that will apply force to the palm side of the hand, at the level of the knuckles (MCP joints) (see diagrams **s-33**, **s-34**, and **s-35**).

Precautions

During the stretch, it is important to keep the finger and hand joints straight,

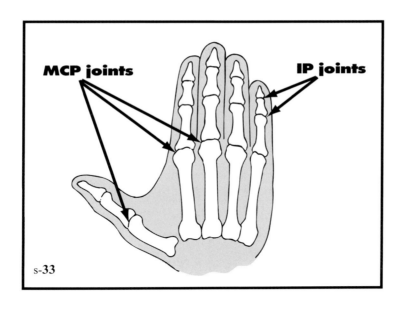

MCP joints

IP joints

s-33

MCP and IP joints

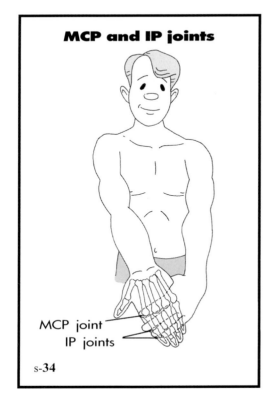

MCP joint
IP joints

s-34

forearm stretch

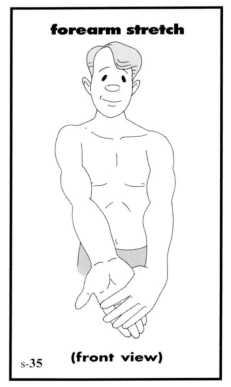

s-35 **(front view)**

without bending them backwards and stressing them into hyperextension. The finger (interphalangeal *IP*) joints, and knuckle (metacarpophalangeal *MCP*) joint of each finger can be stabilized using the fingers of the other hand. Be sure to keep the shoulders relaxed.

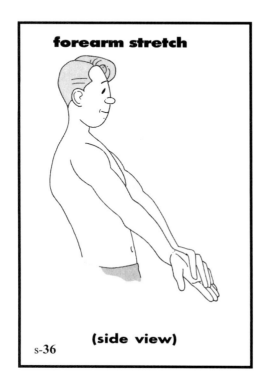

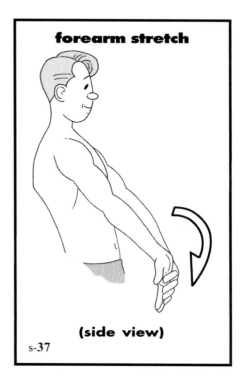

Stretch

The stretch is performed as pressure is applied at the level of the MCP joints in a direction towards the elbow of the hand being stretched (see diagrams **s-36** and **s-37**).

Relaxation/Breathing

Using relaxation breathing techniques, focus on relaxing the neck, both shoulders and the arm, forearm, and hand. Remember to inhale gently and exhale through the mouth, with a conscious puff of the lips. As the forearm

176

muscles relax, the wrist will bend backwards to take up the slack of the relaxing muscles. Do not move beyond what will take up the slack. Slower motion and mindful relaxation will result in deeper levels of stretching. When the wrist and forearm stop releasing, or after 30–45 seconds, gently release the hand and relax.

Recovery

To recover from this stretch, let the arm fall to the side.

Repeat the exercise on the other side if needed. A healthy arm does not need to be stretched as often as the arm with symptoms of pain or carpal tunnel syndrome.

COMBINATION STRETCH

This stretch lengthens the anterior musculature and fascia of the entire arm and forearm at one time. Specifically, this technique works the biceps, forearm, and hand. When the entire length of fascia is stretched at one time, it may appear that the tissue is tighter than had been thought. If there is not enough flexibility to stretch with this technique, the biceps and forearm may first need to be worked on separately (see pages 167 and 174).

▶POSITION

This stretch is performed in a standing position. It can be performed with the hand held against any upright surface. The hand is braced against the wall with the fingers directed upward. Muscles of the shoulder and arm should be kept relaxed and limp. Rotate the arm so that the front side of the elbow joint is pointed downwards as much as possible (see diagram **s-38**).

Precautions

There is a tendency to hold the arm up with the shoulder muscles, and to keep the elbow straight by contracting the triceps muscle. Keep the shoulder

and arm musculature limp and the
shoulder relaxed.

Stretch

The stretch occurs with a
combined motion as the body is
rotated away from the wall. To
increase the level of the stretch,
the hip can be moved slowly and
gently further from the wall (see
diagram **s-38**).

Relaxation/Breathing

Using relaxation breathing
techniques, focus on relaxing the
neck, shoulder, arm, forearm, and
hand. Remember to inhale gently
and exhale through the mouth, with
a conscious puff of the lips. As the
upper extremity muscles relax,
gently and slowly rotate the
body away from the supported
arm. If more stretch is needed,
gently and slowly move the
hip further away from the wall.
Do not move beyond what will
take up the slack of the relaxing
muscles. Slower motion and
mindful relaxation will result in
deeper levels of stretching.

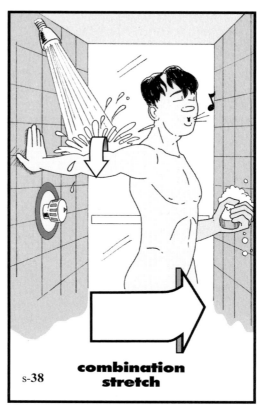

s-38 **combination
stretch**

*With the hand pressed toward the
wall and the fingers pointing upward,
the straight elbow can be rotated so that
it faces upward or downward. The arm
and forearm can be more limp and
relaxed if the arm is rotated as
in the diagram.*

It is easier to relax these muscles with application of moist heat. Try the first stretch of the day while standing in a hot shower with the water running on the upper arm and biceps area.

During this stretch, it is possible to feel a burning discomfort in the arm, forearm, and hand. Further relaxation will allow this feeling to peak and then soften as the muscles and fascia release. Breathe and relax to lessen these sensations before proceeding with moving to stretch further.

Recovery

Move the hip closer to the wall, turn toward facing the wall, and then simply lower the arm and hand.

Repeat the exercise on the other side if needed. A healthy arm should be stretched once per day and does not need to be stretched as often as an arm with symptoms of pain or carpal tunnel syndrome.

TRANSVERSE CARPAL LIGAMENT

The transverse carpal ligament overlies the carpal tunnel or canal through the wrist. This ligament is cut during carpal tunnel surgery to make more room in the canal. Stretching the ligament can also make more room in the canal. The ligament is very tough and will not stretch far. Sometimes the stretch itself can be difficult to feel. Fortunately, a little stretch can be very effective because a small amount of lengthening will translate into significantly more space in the carpal canal. This stretch requires the assistance of a partner, and will be most helpful if it can be done once or twice per day.

⟳POSITION

The person whose wrist is being stretched can be seated in a chair with the affected wrist resting in the lap in a palm up position. The partner holds this wrist with both hands, thumbs on each side of the palm. The fingertips are placed under the middle of the wrist bones (see Position #3, diagrams

s-39). The thumbs of each hand are placed on the palm side of the wrist, one on each side (see Positions #1 and #2 in diagram **s-39** and diagram **s-40**).

Precautions

When force is applied by one person to work on another, it is important that this force be applied gradually and firmly. As the tissues release, maintain steady and firm pressure.

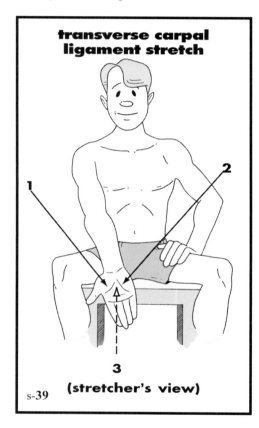

transverse carpal
ligament stretch

(stretcher's view)

s-39

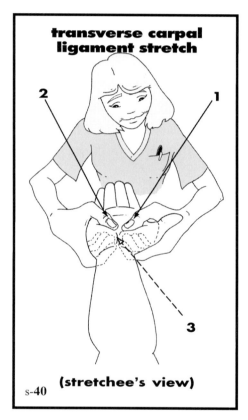

transverse carpal
ligament stretch

(stretchee's view)

s-40

Stretch

The stretch is performed by pushing upward with the fingertips and downward with the thumb tips. This will spread and lengthen the transverse carpal ligament. Slowly increase the force and pressure applied, and then

180

continue the pressure for approximately 30–60 seconds while the person being stretched performs the breathing and relaxation techniques.

Relaxation/Breathing

Using relaxation breathing techniques, focus on relaxing the entire shoulder, upper extremity, and hand. Remember to inhale gently and exhale through the mouth, with a conscious puff of the lips. As the ligament relaxes, the partner should maintain firm pressure with both hands and feel the ligament stretch. Firm pressure and mindful relaxation will result in deeper levels of stretching.

Recovery

When the procedure is complete, pressure is released gradually and gently.

THUMB (THENAR AND ADDUCTOR)

The muscles between the thumb and index finger curl the thumb into the palm and pinch the thumb to the other four fingers. Trigger points in these muscles cause pain in the thumb joints, hand, and fifth finger. Thumb joint pain is often attributed to arthritis. Fortunately, even when there is arthritis in the joint, the pain can be significantly decreased by stretching and massaging these muscles. To stretch these muscles, the thumb must be moved away from the index finger and hand.

This stretch exercise has two basic objectives. The first is to stretch the muscles that move the thumb (thenar and first web space). The other objective is to stretch the transverse carpal ligament (see pages 166 and 179). One of the thumb muscles (flexor pollicus longus) attaches to the transverse carpal ligament, and inserts into the last thumb bone (distal phalanx). This stretch position uses the attachments of the flexor tendon to indirectly stretch the transverse carpal ligament.

In addition, this technique will stretch a significant portion of the fascia of the hand, decreasing tension across the palm.

▬▶POSITION

Hold the thumb firmly with the fingers of the opposite hand so the stretching force can be applied as closely as possible to the MCP joint (where the thumb meets the hand). The hand being stretched should be in a palm up position and the wrist should be limp and dorsiflexed or bent backwards (see diagram **s-41**).

Precautions

During this stretch, it is important to keep the two thumb joints straight, without stressing them into hyperextension. The IP (interphalangeal) joint

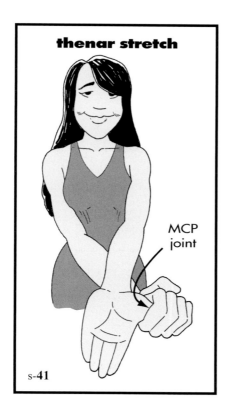

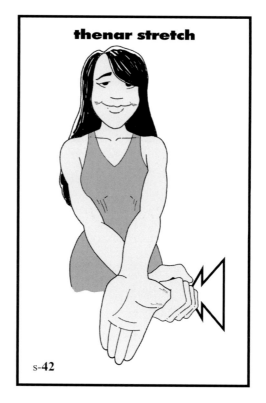

(mid-thumb) and the MCP (metacarpalphanyngeal) joint (where the thumb meets your hand) can be stabilized using the fingers of the other hand (as shown by positioning of the right hand in diagrams **s-41** and **s-42**). MCP and IP joints illustrated on page 175.

Stretch

The stretch is performed by gently and firmly applying pressure to pull the thumb metacarpal back toward the elbow of the same hand (see diagram **s-42**).

Relaxation/Breathing

Using relaxation breathing techniques, focus on relaxing the shoulders, forearm and hand. Remember to inhale gently and exhale through the mouth, with a conscious puff of the lips. As the thumb muscles relax, guide the thumb away from the index finger, taking up the slack in the relaxing muscles. Do not move beyond what will take up the slack of the relaxing muscles. A little bit of motion is a lot of stretch for these muscles. Slower motion and mindful relaxation will result in deeper levels of stretching.

Recovery

When the hand stops releasing, or after 30–45 seconds, gently release the grip around the thumb.

FOREARM (TENNIS ELBOW)

There are several muscles on the top (dorsal) side of the forearm that contribute to pain in the forearm and wrist, as well as the pain of tennis elbow. These include the wrist extensors (extensor carpi radialis and ulnaris), and finger extensors (extensor digitorum). Contraction of these muscles extends the wrist and uncurls the fingers. Repetitive use of these muscles is associated with repetitive strain injuries of the forearm and wrist, as well

stretch

183

as tennis elbow. Frequent breaks and stretching through the day can improve symptoms. To stretch these muscles, the elbow is held straight, and the wrist and then the fingers are curled in the direction of the palm.

⟶POSITION 1 (example left wrist– reverse instructions for the right wrist)

This stretch can be performed in a standing or sitting position. Both arms are placed down and in front of the body with the elbows straight and the palms facing back toward the body. The hand of the arm being stretched is held inside the other hand (see diagram **s-43**).

Precautions

This stretch is performed in stages, and each stage should be completed before progressing to the next. It may take several weeks for the forearm to loosen enough so that all stages may be completed and the muscles are fully stretched. Do not progress to the next stage before the previous stage is fully

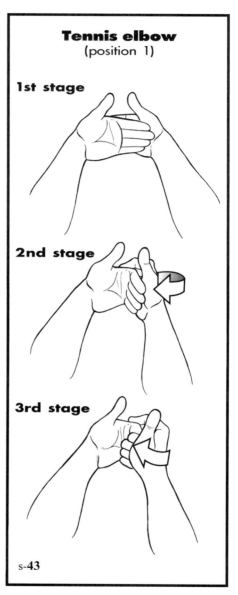

Tennis elbow
(position 1)

1st stage

2nd stage

3rd stage

s-43

stretched. The forearm and hand of the arm being stretched must be totally limp. All the work is done with the other hand. Do not use the muscles of the forearm being stretched to do any of the work of bending the wrist or fingers. Keep the elbow straight, and the shoulders relaxed. A little motion results in a big stretch.

Stretch

The **first** stage of this stretch is to fully bend the wrist with the other hand. The **second** stage is to hold the wrist fully flexed and start to bend the fingers at the knuckle. With the wrist and knuckles fully flexed, the **third** stage is to curl the fingers and bend them towards the palm (see diagram **s-43**).

Relaxation/Breathing

Using relaxation breathing techniques, focus on relaxing both shoulders, forearm, and hand. Remember to inhale gently and exhale through the mouth, with a conscious puff of the lips. As the forearm muscles relax, allow the wrist to bend. After the wrist is fully bent, apply a gentle force to the base of the fingers so that the knuckles flex. Do not move beyond what will take up the slack of the relaxing muscles. When this stage is complete, then apply gentle pressure to the fingers so they start to bend. This part will make the slowest progress. A little bit of motion is a lot of stretch for these muscles. Slower motion and mindful relaxation will result in deeper levels of stretching.

Recovery

When the forearm stops releasing, or after 45–90 seconds, gently release the hold on the hand and allow the arms to drop to the sides (standing) or rest on the lap (sitting).

⇒POSITION 2
(example left wrist-
reverse instructions for the right wrist)

Stand or sit with the elbows straight and the arms in front of the body with the palms facing the body. Cross the right hand over the left hand, rotating the forearms so that the palms are together. Interlock the fingers of both hands. Leave the left elbow straight and the left arm and forearm totally limp (see diagram **s-44**).

Precautions

This stretch should be performed gently and slowly, keeping the shoulders as relaxed as possible.

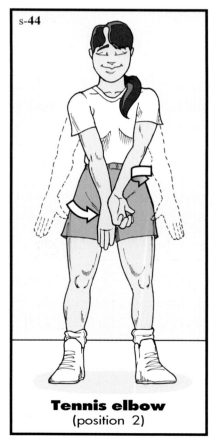

Tennis elbow
(position 2)

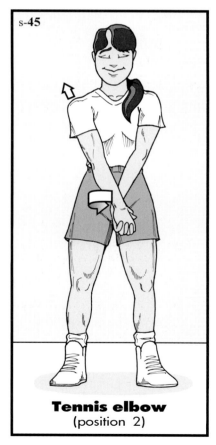

Tennis elbow
(position 2)

Stretch

This stretch starts with straightening the right wrist. Next, push down and away from the body, pulling the left wrist being stretched. Lastly, slowly rotate the right forearm outwards (toward the right) so that the left forearm internally rotates (see diagram **s-45**).

Relaxation/Breathing

Using relaxation breathing techniques, focus on relaxing the left forearm and hand, and only allow a small amount of movement with each breath. Remember to inhale gently and exhale through the mouth, with a conscious puff of the lips. Do not move beyond what will take up the slack of the relaxing muscles. A little bit of motion is a lot of stretch for these muscles. Slower motion and mindful relaxation will result in deeper levels of stretching.

Recovery

When this stretch is finished relax both arms and let go of the hands.

HAND and FINGER

The muscles inside the hands move the knuckles and the fingers. The lumbricales flex the knuckles and straighten the finger joints. The belly of these muscles is located between the bones of the hand, from the wrist to the knuckles. Pain from trigger points in these muscles goes to the knuckles, fingers, and the finger joints. To stretch these muscles, the knuckles have to be straight while the fingers curl.

➠POSITION 1
(example left wrist–
reverse instructions for the right wrist)

This stretch is easily performed in a seated position. Place both hands on the lap, palm up, holding the left hand being stretched with the right hand. Place the pad of the working right index finger on the back of the knuckle of the finger being stretched. Curl the left finger being stretched with the working right thumb on the left finger nail (see diagram **s-46**).

Precautions

Swelling of the finger joints may cause pain when these joints are flexed. Stop this stretch when this pain occurs.

Stretch

This stretch starts with hyperextending the knuckle of the left hand, bending it back with pressure of the right thumb. The back of the stretching left knuckle is stabilized with the index finger of the right hand. After the knuckle is extended (bent backwards), push with the right thumb on the left fingernail, bending the joints of the left finger (see diagram **s-46**).

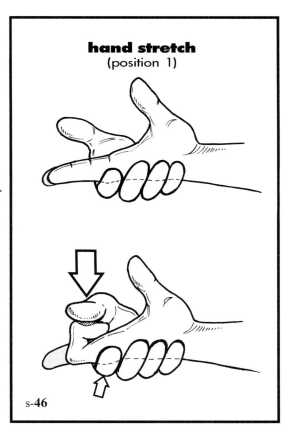

hand stretch
(position 1)

s-46

Relaxation/Breathing

Using relaxation breathing techniques, focus on relaxing both shoulders, and the arm and hand being stretched. It should take a few breaths for the knuckle to bend backward and then the finger joints to stretch. Remember to inhale gently and exhale through the mouth, with a conscious puff of the lips. As the hand and finger muscles relax, bend the finger joints further, taking up the slack in the relaxing muscles. Do not move beyond what will take up the slack of the relaxing muscles. A little bit of motion is a lot of stretch for these muscles. Slower motion and mindful relaxation will result in deeper levels of stretching.

Recovery

To recover from this stretch, gently relax the right hand doing the work and let go.

⟶POSITION 2

Another position for stretching the muscles in the hand can be done with both hands at the same time. This stretch is easily performed in a seated position. With both hands comfortably in front of the body at belly level, place the fingertips together—thumb to thumb, and finger to finger (see diagram **s-47**). It does not matter whether the forearms are rotated so that the thumbs are pointed up or down. The stretch should be tried with the hands rotated in various directions. Feel for comfort or for the best feeling stretch.

Precautions

Pain or swelling in the knuckle or finger joint may prevent this stretch from being done. If these joints are painful after the stretch, try not stretching as far, even if no stretch is felt at the time. Be gentle. The arm muscles are much stronger than the finger joints.

Stretch

This stretch occurs as the palms are pressed together, straightening the fingers and the palms.

Relaxation/Breathing

Using relaxation breathing techniques, focus on relaxing both forearms and hands. Remember to inhale gently and exhale through the mouth, with a conscious puff of the lips. Keep the upper back, head, and neck upright. As the hand and finger muscles relax, continue to apply gentle pressure pushing the palms together. Do not move beyond what will take up the slack in the relaxing muscles. Slower motion and mindful relaxation will result in deeper levels of stretching.

Recovery

To recover from this stretch, simply let go and allow the hands to drop to a relaxed position.

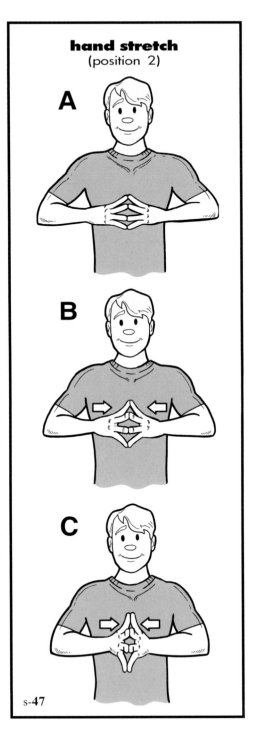

hand stretch
(position 2)

A

B

C

s-47

LOWER BACK

There are several muscles that contribute to lower back pain. These include muscles along the spine from the pelvis to the scalp (paraspinal), deep muscles of the lower back (quadratus lumborum), muscles of the flank (lower latissimus and abdominal obliques), gluteal muscles (gluteus maximus, medius, and minimus), and muscles of the pelvic floor (coccygeus and levator ani).

PARASPINAL MUSCLES

The long paraspinal muscles inter-link from the neck to the lower back like the links on a metal wristwatch band. They act primarily to straighten the spine and help with rotation. To stretch these muscles, the spine has to be curved forwards. It is most effective to stretch the entire column at the same time.

⫸POSITION

Start seated with your feet flat on the floor. Place your hands comfortably on the top of the thighs or knees (see diagrams **s-48** and **s-49**).

Precautions

Keep this stretch slow and gentle. The entire body weight should be supported with the hands so that the back muscles can be totally limp. Allow only a small amount of stretching motion with each breath. **Do not stretch into pain or through pain.** During recovery, uncoil the spine and do not raise the head until after the upper back is fully upright. Lifting the head earlier will tighten the muscles of the entire spine.

Stretch

The stretch starts with letting the neck bend and the head drop straight

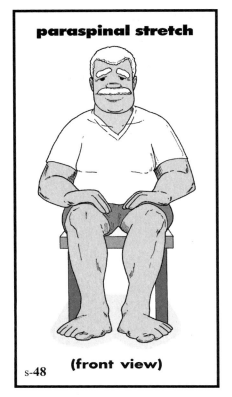

paraspinal stretch

s-48 **(front view)**

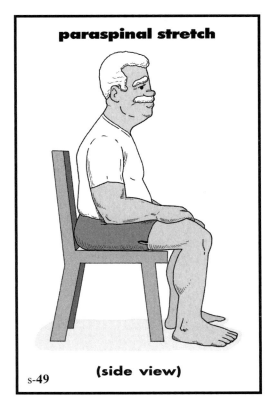

paraspinal stretch

s-49 **(side view)**

forward. After a few breaths, the head will come to rest with its own weight balanced by soft tissue tension in the back of the neck. The next motion is to gradually slump the shoulders forward, supporting the entire weight of the upper body with the arms and hands. The body should continue to fall gently forward, until there is no more muscle slack or the chest has come to rest between the thighs (see diagrams **s-50** and **s-51**). Remember to inhale gently and exhale through the mouth, with a conscious puff of the lips. Do not move beyond what will take up the slack of the relaxing muscles. Slower motion and mindful relaxation will result in deeper levels of stretching.

Relaxation/Breathing

Using relaxation breathing and techniques, focus on relaxing the neck, shoulders, and entire back. It will take at least the first three breaths for the head to drop. It should take at least seven to ten more breaths for the body to come forward and down. The muscles of the neck and back need to be as limp as possible, and should not be contracting to support the body's weight. As with other stretches, the forward stretching motion should take place during exhalation and relaxation.

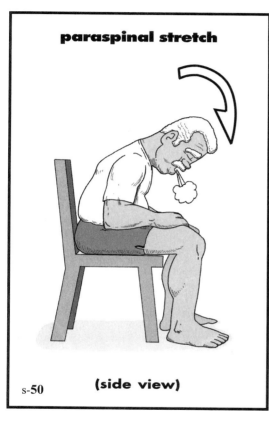

paraspinal stretch

s-50 **(side view)**

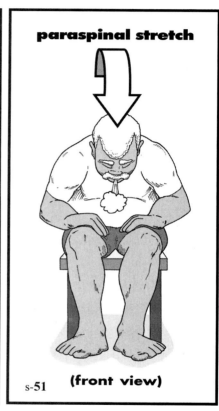

paraspinal stretch

s-51 **(front view)**

Recovery

To come out of this stretch, slowly uncoil the spine. Start by pushing downward with your hands to raise up, keeping the neck limp and the head hanging forward. Uncoil the spine, and when the lower back is erect, release the slump of the shoulders and straighten the upper back. Keep the neck limp and let the head continue to hang until the upper back is erect. Finally,

193

raise the head to an upright position.

QUADRATUS LUMBORUM

This muscle tilts and twists the lower back. Stretching this muscle requires twisting the lower body. *A stretching session **should never begin or end** with such a twist of the body.* Therefore, be sure to perform a straight paraspinal muscle stretch (above) before and after performing this stretch.

Ⅲ➡POSITION

Start this stretch lying down on one side. Then bend the top hip and knee approximately 90 degrees, resting this knee on the mat. Tuck the lower shoulder forward and rest the lower hand upon this knee (see diagram **s-52**).

Precautions

Do not try to actively twist the lower back and force the stretch. The muscles of the lower back must fully relax and not contract to assist with this stretch. If an additional gentle force is needed, rest the upper hand on the buttocks, and gently push forward and downward toward the feet (lying on the left side, this would be the right hand). **Before rolling over to stretch the other side, be sure to bring the shoulders and hips back into parallel alignment. Do not try to get up or turn over while the shoulders are open and the lower back is rotated.**

Stretch

This stretch starts with moving the top hand and arm to a position behind the body. The upper shoulder will open up and the upper body will start to twist. As the arm comes over the body, turn the head to follow the arm and look toward the hand. The stretch continues as the weight of the arm leads the upper body to twist (see diagram **s-53**). If additional force is desired, rest the top hand on the upper buttocks and gently push forward and

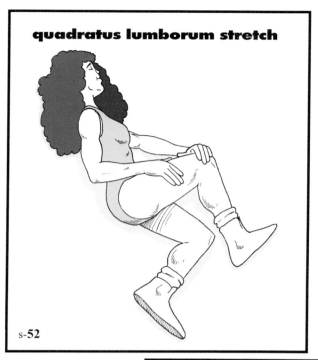

quadratus lumborum stretch

s-52

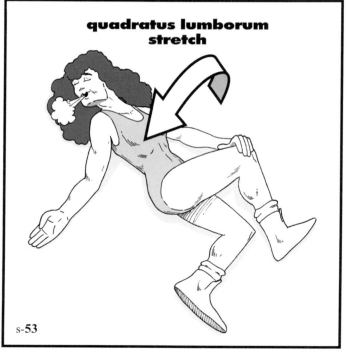

quadratus lumborum stretch

s-53

downward toward the feet.

Relaxation/Breathing

Using relaxation breathing techniques, focus on relaxing the muscles of the lower back and hip, and barely move with each breath. Remember to inhale gently and exhale through the mouth, with a conscious puff of the lips. As the lower back relaxes, allow the weight of the arm to provide a twisting force to stretch this lower back muscle, and move only to take up the slack as the muscle relaxes. Slower motion and mindful relaxation will result in deeper levels of stretching. With successive breaths, gently allow the body to twist further.

Recovery

To end the stretch, bring the upper arm to the front of the body, face forward, and close the upper shoulder so that the shoulders are square with the hips. Once the upper body is aligned with the lower body, you can turn to the other side or to get up. **Do not try to get up or turn over while the shoulders are open and the lower back is rotated.**

Turn by rolling over the back or over the abdomen, whichever is more comfortable.

LOWER LATISSIMUS

This muscle pulls the shoulder girdle towards the hip, and also internally rotates and moves the upper arm backwards and towards the body. Stretching this muscle requires stabilizing the pelvis and allowing the arm and shoulder to move towards the head.

These stretches will lengthen and relax all the muscles along the side of the body, from the waist to the underarm. They can be performed effectively in both standing and lying down positions.

⟹POSITION 1

For the standing position stretch, stand sideways and approximately 6 inches away from a wall or other solid support. The arms should be raised overhead and the body should have a slight bend towards the wall (see diagram **s-54**).

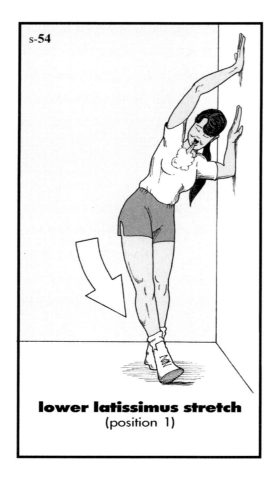

s-54

lower latissimus stretch
(position 1)

Precautions

This stretch does not require much motion. A little bit goes a long way. Do not allow your hip to drop very far at first. During recovery, do not use the muscles that were just stretched to straighten your body. Be sure to follow the recovery directions carefully.

Stretch

The stretch is performed by bending the outside knee and allowing the hip to fall. To stretch further, the outer leg can be moved out in front as shown. The stretch will be felt more to the back or to the side, depending on the position of the pelvis. If the pelvis is slightly tucked during the process (pubic bone pushed forward a little), the stretch will focus more on the muscles that insert into the posterior pelvis (see diagram **s-54**). The lower back can also be slightly extended during the stretch (pubic bone pushed backward a little), causing the stretch to focus more on the muscles that insert into the anterior part of the pelvis.

Relaxation/Breathing

Using relaxation breathing techniques, focus on relaxing the muscles of the entire side of the body from the shoulder to the hip, and only allow a little bit of movement with each breath. Remember to inhale gently and exhale through the mouth, with a conscious puff of the lips. As the muscles of the side of the body relax and lengthen, the hip will gently lower. Four or five deep breaths will usually be enough to allow this muscle group to relax and the stretch to be effective. Do not move beyond what will take up the slack of the relaxing muscles. Slower motion and mindful relaxation will result in deeper levels of stretching.

Recovery

To end this stretch, straighten the outside knee and push the upper body away from the wall using the arms. When both legs are evenly bearing weight, the stretch is over.

Then the other side can be lengthened in a similar fashion. *This stretch can be easily performed in the shower.*

⁞⟶POSITION 2

These muscles can also be stretched in a lying down position. To make this easier, it is best to be on an elevated surface such as a bed. Lie on one side near the bottom of the bed with the lower knee bent. The upper leg should be relaxed, with the leg resting on the edge of the bed. This will place the body in a position that starts to open and stretch the upper side. Place the arms above the head with the lower hand holding the upper wrist (see diagram **s-55**).

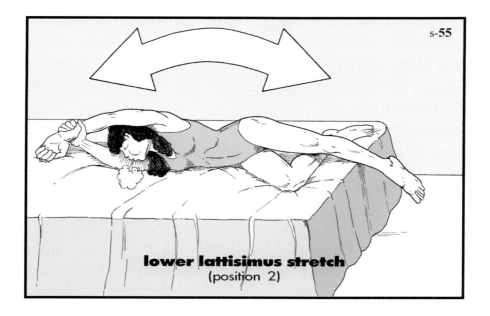

s-55

lower lattisimus stretch
(position 2)

Precautions

This is a very gentle stretch and does not require much motion to be helpful. **Do not pull at either end of the body—the hand above or the leg below**. Also, do not continue this stretch for more than five or six breaths. Lastly, finish the recovery as described below before turning to the other side or getting up.

199

Stretch

The stretch is performed by allowing the pelvis to move away from the lower ribs (see diagram **s-55**).

Relaxation/Breathing

Using relaxation breathing techniques, focus on relaxing the entire side of the body from the shoulder to the hip, and allow only a little bit of movement with each breath. Remember to inhale gently and exhale through the mouth, with a conscious puff of the lips. As the muscles of the side relax, gently hold the wrist, and let the weight of the upper leg pull the pelvis away from the ribs. Do not move beyond what will take up the slack in the relaxing muscles. Slower motion and mindful relaxation will result in deeper levels of stretching.

Recovery

To finish the stretch bend both hips, tuck the knees towards the chest, and feel the pelvis begin to level before turning over to lengthen the other side.

RECTUS ABDOMINUS

This muscle flexes the spine and especially the lower back. Stretching this muscle requires some degree of arching the spine. This is minimized by holding the muscle in a small degree of stretch and then using the hands and fingers to lengthen the muscle and fascia.

This stretch will lengthen and relax the muscle and fascia that goes down the middle of the abdomen from the lower ribs to the pubis.

⟫➡POSITION

Start this stretch lying down on your back. If abdominal muscles are tight or the lower back cannot tolerate a slight backwards bend into extension,

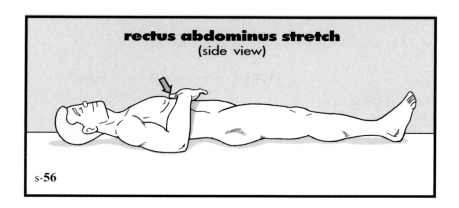

rectus abdominus stretch
(side view)

s-56

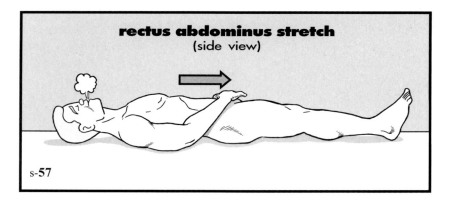

rectus abdominus stretch
(side view)

s-57

it will be best to lie flat on the bed or floor (see diagram **s-56**). Those who are more flexible can lie on a bed and let the lower legs hang down off the edge. This will put a slight stretch on the rectus muscle and slightly arch the lower spine.

Precautions

Some people get relief from lower back pain when their lower back is positioned in extension. Others find that their lower back pain worsens. This stretch should first be tried with the body and legs lying flat and at the same level (see diagram **s-57**). If additional stretch is needed, try first to dangle the legs off the edge of the bed at the knee. Aggravation of lower back pain

201

this increased extension will mean that most of the stretching action should be done by the hands and fingers.

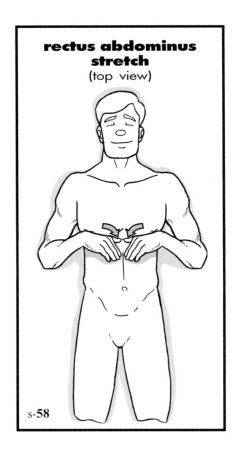

rectus abdominus
stretch
(top view)

s-58

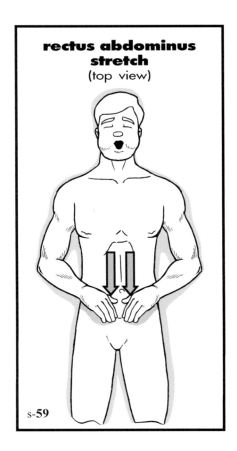

rectus abdominus
stretch
(top view)

s-59

Stretch

This stretch starts with placing the hands in the middle of the body and just below the sternum (see diagrams **s-56** and **s-58**). Push gently into the abdomen with either the fingertips or the sides of the thumbs. This inward push "engages" the muscle and fascia. The stretch occurs as the fingers or thumbs continue to slide down to the pubic bone (see diagrams **s-57** and **s-59**).

Relaxation/Breathing

Using relaxation breathing techniques, focus on relaxing the abdomen and lower back. Thinking about relaxing the shoulders, arms, and hands will help keep them from tensing. It should take a few breaths for the hands to slide all the way down to the pelvis. Remember to inhale gently and exhale through the mouth, with a conscious puff of the lips. As the abdominal muscles relax, continue to slide the hands down toward the pelvis. Do not slide the hands quickly. Slower motion and mindful relaxation will result in deeper levels of stretching.

Recovery

To recover from this stretch, gently relax the hands and ease up on pushing into the abdomen and pubic bone. Then roll onto the side or stomach and get up.

GLUTEUS/PIRIFORMIS

The gluteal and piriformis muscles work together to move the thigh out to the side and behind the body. They also rotate the hip joint outwards. Stretching these muscles involves a combination of bringing the thigh forward, across and out from the body, and rotating the hip joint in and out. These muscles get injured during twisting and lifting, running, and kicking out and back.

⯈POSITION 1

One of the simplest positions for stretching the piriformis and gluteal muscles is seated on a chair. The technique is very similar to that used for the long paraspinal muscles of the back (see pages 191–193). Once seated in the chair, lift one leg and place the ankle area upon the opposite knee. Rest the ankle where it is most comfortable. Then place one hand on the elevated knee and the other on the ankle for support (see diagram **s-60**).

gluteus/piriformis stretch
(position 1)

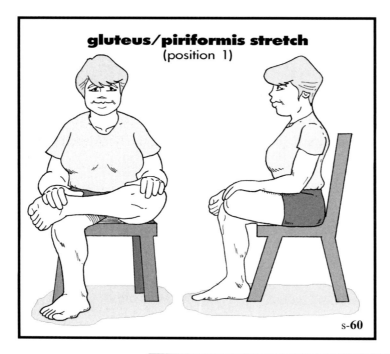

s-60

gluteus/piriformis stretch
(position 1)

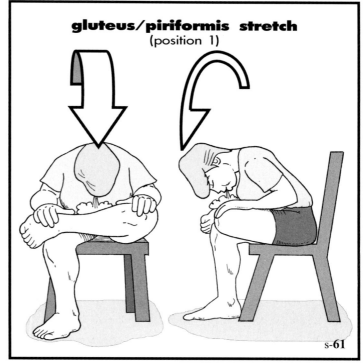

s-61

Precautions

Keep this stretch slow and gentle. The weight of the upper body should be totally supported with the hands so that the back muscles can be totally limp. Allow only a small amount of stretching motion with each breath. **Do not stretch into pain or through pain.** During recovery, do not raise the head until after the upper back is fully upright. Lifting the head earlier will tighten the muscles of the entire spine—from neck to sacrum. For this reason, resist the tendency to interrupt this stretch before completing the recovery to upright posture.

Stretch

The stretch starts with letting the neck bend and the head drop straight forward. After a few breaths, the head will come to rest with its own weight balanced by soft tissue tension in the back of the neck. Then allow the body to lean forward, supporting the weight with the hands pressing on the knee and ankle (see diagram **s-61**). Slowly continue to lower the body forward, until there is no more slack or until the chest has come to rest between the thighs.

As the body comes forward, the stretch (and sometimes a burning sensation) will be felt in the buttocks and around the side and back of the upper thigh. With successive breaths, this discomfort will subside, allowing more motion and greater stretch.

Relaxation/Breathing

Using relaxation breathing techniques, focus on relaxing the muscles of the neck, lower back, and hip, moving no further than about 15 degrees with each exhalation. Remember to inhale gently and exhale through the mouth, with a conscious puff of the lips. As the hip and lower back muscles relax, slowly allow the head to fall forward until the neck is limp. Then allow the body to lean forward, supporting the weight with the hands pressing

stretch

on the knee and ankle. As the body comes forward, the stretch (and sometimes a burning sensation) will be felt in the buttocks and around the side and back of the upper thigh. With successive breaths, this discomfort will subside, allowing more motion and greater stretch. Slower motion and mindful relaxation will result in deeper levels of stretching.

Recovery

To come out of this stretch, slowly uncoil the spine. Start by pushing with the hands to raise up, leaving the neck limp and the head hanging forward. When the lower back is erect, release the slump of the shoulders and straighten the upper back. Keep the neck limp and let the head continue to hang until the upper back is erect. Finally, finish uncoiling the spine by raising the head to an upright position.

▰▸POSITION 2

These muscles can also be stretched in a standing position. This may be important for stretching at work when sitting is not possible, and during other physical activities. Start by standing and leaning back, resting the buttocks on an object of table height. Then lift one leg up and pull the knee and ankle toward the chest (see diagram **s-62**).

Precautions

This stretch is performed while balancing on one foot, and leaning/ resting and supporting the buttocks. Be careful to be well supported and not to lose balance. A large belly and difficulty balancing will make this stretch position extremely difficult, and perhaps unsafe.

Stretch

While holding the knee with one hand, grip the ankle with the opposite hand and lift the ankle upwards. This will rotate the hip outwards. Next, pull toward the chest with both hands and move the thigh, knee, and ankle toward the chest. The stretch will be felt in the buttocks and outer thigh (see diagram **s-63**).

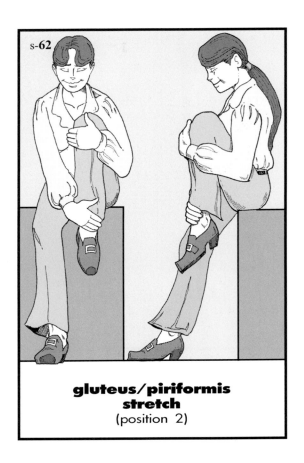

**gluteus/piriformis
stretch**
(position 2)

Relaxation/Breathing

Using relaxation breathing techniques, focus on relaxing the hip and lower back. As the hip muscles relax, give a firm and gentle pull with both hands, bringing the knee and leg toward the chest. Do not move beyond what will take up the slack in the relaxing muscles. Remember to inhale gently and exhale through the mouth, with a conscious puff of the lips. Slower motion and mindful relaxation will result in deeper levels of stretching.

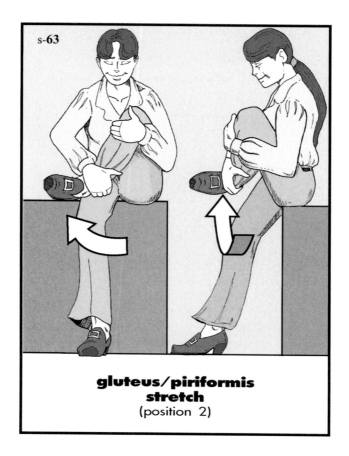

**gluteus/piriformis
stretch**
(position 2)

Recovery

To end this stretch, keep the back and body upright, and slowly lower the knee and ankle to waist level before letting go with the hands.

⇒POSITION 3

The most effective stretch for gluteal and outer thigh muscles is performed lying down on the back. This position also deeply stretches the fascia of the outside of the hip and lower extremity.

To start this stretch, a rope or towel (a jump rope with knots to help grip may be best) is placed under the arch of the foot and held with both hands. The hip and thigh are kept limp and relaxed as the hands pull on the rope and lift the leg and foot 12–18 inches above the floor (see diagram **s-64**).

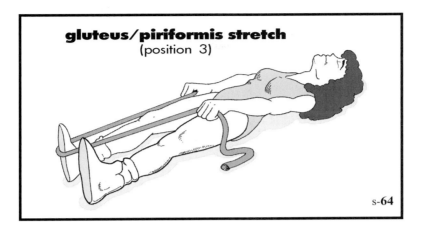

gluteus/piriformis stretch
(position 3)

s-64

Precautions

This stretch requires a moderate level of upper body strength. It should be done only with caution by people who have neck and upper body pain Stretch positions should not be held long enough to fatigue the upper body, hands, or arms. Do not stretch into pain or beyond the edge of numbness.

If pain is felt on the inside of the upper thigh and hip during this stretch, it is likely that the adductor and iliopsoas muscles (upper and inner thigh)

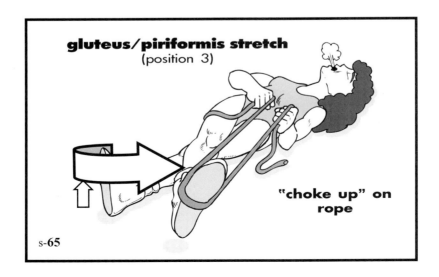

gluteus/piriformis stretch
(position 3)

"choke up" on
rope

s-65

are contracting. This can be avoided by focusing more on relaxing these muscles and holding the entire weight of the leg with the rope.

Stretch

While holding the rope with both hands, lift and guide the leg across the body to the opposite side. If the leg moves far enough, "choke up" on the rope and take up the slack so that the elbows can be kept relaxed, and extended (see diagram **s-65**).

Relaxation/Breathing

Using relaxation breathing techniques, focus on relaxing the buttocks, groin, and thigh. Do not tense the upper shoulders, and move the leg no more than about 15 degrees with each exhalation. Remember to inhale gently and exhale through the mouth, with a conscious puff of the lips. As the hip and thigh muscles relax, gently pull on the rope and lead it sideways to guide the leg across the body. Do not move beyond what will take up the slack of the relaxing buttocks and thigh muscles. You may feel temporary numbness in the leg and foot. With successive breaths, this discomfort will subside, allowing more motion and greater stretch. Slower motion and mindful relaxation will result in deeper levels of stretching.

Recovery

Slowly relax the rope and allow the leg to cross back over the body and rest next to the other leg. Keep the hip totally relaxed, with all the weight of the leg held by the rope.

LOWER EXTREMITY

There are several hip and thigh muscles that contribute to lower extremity pain. These include muscles of the buttocks (gluteal), muscles of the inside of the pelvis and hip (iliopsoas), muscles of the inside of the hip (adductor), and muscles of the front and back of the thigh (quadriceps and hamstring).

GLUTEAL

The gluteal muscles work together to move the thigh out to the side and behind the body. They also rotate the hip joint outwards. The stretches for these muscles are discussed previously (see pages 203–210).

The gluteal and piriformis muscles work together to move the thigh out to the side and behind the body, and they rotate the hip joint outwards. Stretching these muscles involves a combination of bringing the thigh forward, across and out from the body, and rotating the hip joint in and out. These muscles get injured during twisting and lifting, running and kicking out and back.

HAMSTRING

The hamstring muscles bend the knee and move the thigh backwards. Stretching these muscles involves a combination of straightening the knee and flexing the hip (bending the hip forward). There are three good positions for stretching these muscles: standing, sitting, and lying down. Use the position that allows the best relaxation and most frequent opportunities for stretching. The most important rule to follow with regard to positioning is that the hamstring muscle must be completely relaxed if stretching is to be effective and relatively comfortable.

These muscles are very important when treating lower back pain. Even if there are no thigh pain symptoms, stretching these muscles should be considered.

stretch

211

Hamstring muscles get injured during lifting, running and overstretching especially during play.

⫸POSITION 1

Many people relax best and stretch their hamstrings most effectively when lying on their backs. In this position, the foot and leg are held by a rope or towel placed under the instep of the foot (see diagram **s-66**).

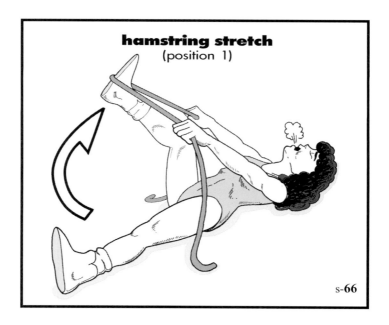

hamstring stretch
(position 1)

s-66

Precautions

This stretch requires a moderate level of upper body strength. It should be done only with caution by people who have neck and upper body pain. Stretch positions should not be held long enough to fatigue the upper body, hands, or arms. Also, do not stretch into pain or beyond the edge of numbness.

Stretch

The stretch occurs as the rope is pulled by the hands and the leg is lifted upward. As this happens, the hands should "choke up" or "take up the slack" on the rope so that the elbows and arms can stay relaxed not flexed (see diagram **s-66**).

When the leg is up in the air, the ankle should be high enough to be perpendicular to the waist, allowing the force of gravity to help perform this stretch. This helps reduce arm fatigue. If the ankle is not raised this far, gravity will pull the leg back towards the floor. Some people will be able to keep their knee straight, and others will have to bend the knee in order to move the leg up this far. If the leg is not moved up this far, gravity will be pulling the leg back toward the floor and the arms will quickly become tired.

Using relaxation breathing techniques, focus on relaxing the hip and thigh, do not tense the upper shoulders, and move very slowly once a gentle pull is felt in the hamstrings. Remember to inhale gently and exhale through the mouth, with a conscious puff of the lips. As the hamstrings relax, gently pull on the rope to guide the leg upward, and move just enough to take up the slack of the relaxing muscles. It is possible to feel temporary numbness in the leg and foot. Do not move beyond what will take up the slack in the relaxing muscles. Slower motion and mindful relaxation will result in deeper levels of stretching.

Recovery

Slowly relax the rope, lower the leg to the mat, and set it to rest next to the other leg. Keep the hip totally relaxed with all the weight of the leg held by the rope.

➡POSITION 2

The hamstrings can also be stretched in a general standing position. Place both feet shoulder-width apart, slowly dropping the head and then the body forward and downward, bending at the waist, arms hanging limp.

Precautions

Balancing in this position can be difficult, so progress slowly and try to maintain control with the feet. **This position should not be performed by a person with lower back pain or herniated disc conditions**. Recovery from this stretch should be carefully performed according to the description below and the diagrams. With extreme caution, this exercise can be done in the shower with the warm water pulsing on the lower back and the back of the thighs.

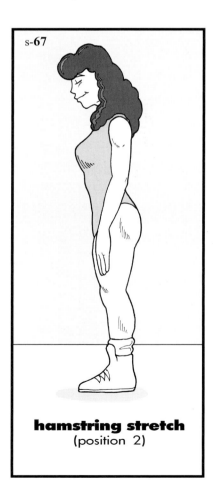

s-67

hamstring stretch
(position 2)

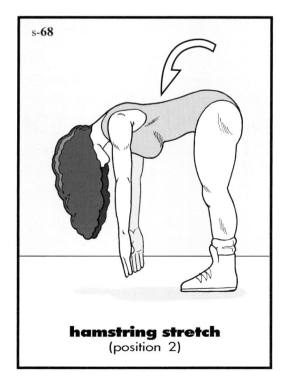

s-68

hamstring stretch
(position 2)

Stretch

The stretch starts by hanging the head toward the feet, rounding the shoulders forward, and starting to lean forward (see diagram **s-67**)—first with the upper body and then gradually with the middle, lower back, and then the hip areas. Allow the arms to just hang from the shoulders and slowly go as far downward as flexibility will permit (see diagram **s-68**).

At first, this stretch will be felt mostly in the upper back and neck, especially if the neck and shoulders are well relaxed and can remain limp. As the back loosens, the body will move forward and the hip and hamstring muscles will start to come under tension. Keep the knees locked. Eventually, it may be possible to totally hang the upper body in a forward bending position, chest against the knees, supported only by the feet.

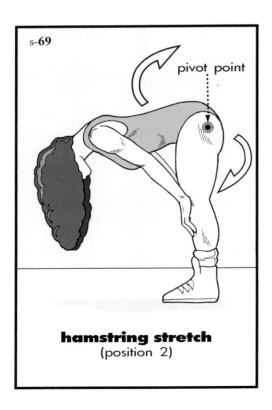

s-**69**

pivot point

hamstring stretch
(position 2)

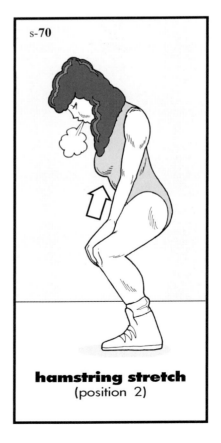

s-**70**

hamstring stretch
(position 2)

stretch

Relaxation/Breathing

Using relaxation breathing techniques, focus on relaxing the neck, shoulders, back, and hamstrings. Remember to inhale gently and exhale through the mouth, with a conscious puff of the lips. As the muscles relax, allow the arms to hang from the shoulders, and slowly allow the upper body to bend farther and lower the hands toward the ground. The shoulders will also relax more as the hands move gently towards the floor. Move slowly enough to maintain balance and do not move farther than what will take up the slack in the relaxing muscles. Slower motion and mindful relaxation will result in deeper levels of stretching.

Recovery

To stand back up, place the hands on the knees (see diagram **s-69**), bend the knees, and then push the body upright with the arms (see diagram **s-70**).

⇒POSITION 3

Another hamstring stretch from a standing position starts with propping one foot on top of a box or step and balancing on the other foot with the hand(s) holding onto something that is about at waist height.

Precautions

Keep the body balanced and the upper body supported with the hands braced on surrounding objects such as a table (see diagram **s-71**).

Stretch

The stretch starts with hanging the head down, rounding the shoulders forward, and starting to lean forward—first with the upper body and then gradually with the middle, lower back, and then the hip areas. As the upper body relaxes and slowly moves forward, a tightening will be felt in the hamstring muscles.

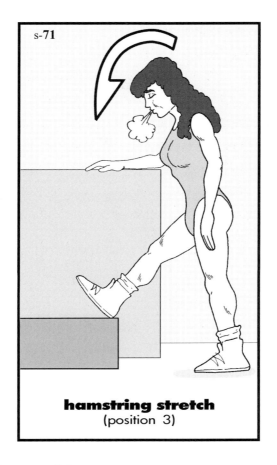

hamstring stretch
(position 3)

Relaxation/Breathing

Using relaxation breathing techniques, focus on relaxing the neck, back, buttocks, and hamstrings. Remember to inhale gently and exhale through the mouth, with a conscious puff of the lips. As the muscles relax, allow the body to lean further forward to apply light pressure to stretch the hamstrings. Do not move beyond what will take up the slack in the relaxing hamstrings. Slower motion and mindful relaxation will result in deeper levels of stretching.

Recovery

At this point, gently lean forward to apply light pressure to the hamstrings for several seconds, and take a few deep and relaxing breaths. Gradually lift and uncoil the spine, vertebrae by vertebrae.

⫸POSITION 4

The hamstring muscles can also be stretched in a seated position, one leg extended with the heel on the floor and the other leg with the foot flat on the floor (see diagram **s-72**).

Precautions

Keep this stretch slow and gentle. The entire body weight should be supported with the hands so that the back muscles can be totally limp. The neck should be kept as limp as possible and the head should "hang." Allow only a small amount of stretching motion with each breath. **Do not stretch into pain or through pain.** During recovery, do not raise the head until after the upper back is fully upright. Lifting the head earlier will tighten the muscles of the entire spine.

Stretch

The stretch starts with hanging the head down (see diagram **s-72),** rounding the shoulders forward, and starting to lean forward—first with the upper body and then gradually the entire back (see diagram **s-73).** As the upper body relaxes and slowly moves forward, a tightening will be felt in the hamstring muscles.

Relaxation/Breathing

Using relaxation breathing techniques, focus on relaxing the neck, back, buttocks, and hamstrings. Remember to inhale gently and exhale through the mouth, with a conscious puff of the lips. As the muscles relax, allow the body to lean further forward to apply light pressure to stretch the hamstrings. Do not move beyond what will take up the slack in the relaxing

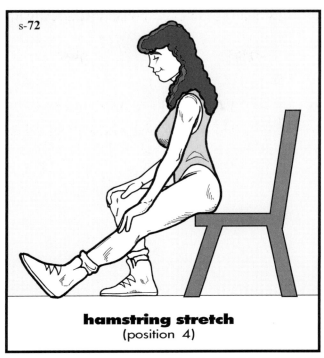

hamstring stretch
(position 4)

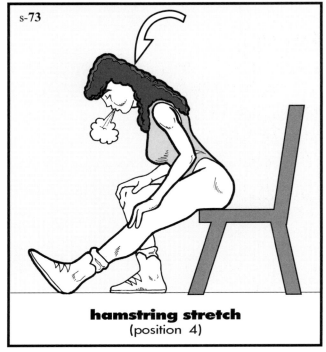

hamstring stretch
(position 4)

hamstrings. Slower motion and mindful relaxation will result in deeper levels of stretching.

Recovery

To come out of this stretch, slowly push with the hands and start to raise up, keeping the neck limp and the head hanging forward. When the lower back is erect, release the slump of the shoulders and straighten the upper back. The neck remains limp and the head continues to hang until the upper back is erect. Finally, the spine "uncoils" and the head is raised last to an upright position.

QUADRICEPS

Contraction of the quadriceps muscles brings the thigh forward (flexes the hip) and straightens (extends) the knee joint. To stretch this muscle, the hip joint must remain straight as the knee is flexed. To stretch even further, extend the hip joint by moving the thigh backwards, before flexing the knee. There are three good positions for stretching these muscles: one standing and two lying down. Position 3 (see pages 224–225) is for people who have more flexibility. Use the position that is best at that moment. The most important rule to follow with regard to positioning is that the quadriceps muscles must be completely relaxed if stretching is to be effective and relatively comfortable.

These muscles are very important when treating hip and knee pain. They also cause numbness in the front of the thigh, even across to the opposite thigh. Even if there are no thigh pain symptoms, stretching these muscles should be considered.

Quadriceps muscles get injured during jumping, running, sudden starts, and kicking forward.

⟶POSITION 1

To perform this stretch in a standing position you must be able to stand and balance on one foot. It is best to hold onto something for balance, and also use this object to apply pressure to the front of the thigh for help with extending the hip joint. Remember that this stretch is more effective if the hip is kept straight or extended. Note that people with very limited flexibility may not be able to keep their hips extended.

Next, grasp the ankle with the hand of the same side (i.e. right hand-right ankle). To get into this position, it is best to kick the heel upward and backward and catch the ankle with the hand (see diagram **s-74**).

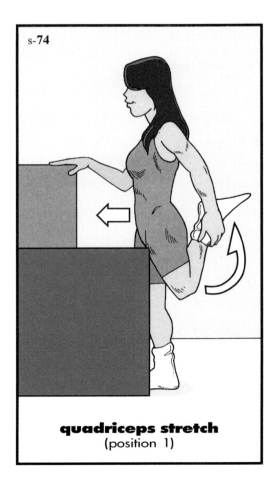

quadriceps stretch
(position 1)

Precautions

Keep the body balanced, using a countertop or other object for support. Use a cabinet or similar object to push the thigh backwards so that the arm and shoulder do not have to do this work. Pulling backwards with the hand to keep the hip straight can cause the upper shoulder and back muscles to spasm. When kicking the ankle up, take care not to injure the hand. Lifting the leg slowly, rather than kicking it up, can cause the hamstring to spasm.

Stretch

Allow the cabinet to push the thigh backward and keep the hip straight. The stretch occurs as the hand pulls the ankle toward the buttocks (see diagram **s-74**).

Relaxation/Breathing

Using relaxation breathing techniques, focus on relaxing the hip and thigh, lifting the ankle only a little bit with each exhalation. Remember to inhale gently and exhale through the mouth, with a conscious puff of the lips. Do not move beyond what will take up the slack in the relaxing muscles. Slower motion and mindful relaxation will result in deeper levels of stretching.

Recovery

To recover from this stretch, gently lower the ankle and let go, allowing the foot to return to the floor. Stand on both feet evenly. Then proceed to stretch the other leg.

⟩POSITION 2

Quadriceps stretching can also be performed in a lying down position, on the side or stomach. The stomach technique may be easiest on a flat surface. A bed or floor will help to keep the hip joint straight. For those who are less flexible, placing a pillow under the hips may be helpful. Bending the knee, grasp the ankle of the leg to be stretched with the same side hand

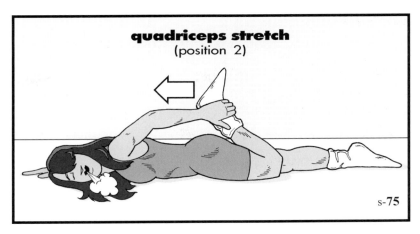

quadriceps stretch
(position 2)

s-75

(see diagram **s-75**).

Alternatively, wrap a strap around the ankle and pull with the hand(s) to bend the knee (see diagram **s-76**). This is the easiest stretch position for less flexible people.

Precautions

Keep the shoulder and upper back as relaxed and comfortable as possible. **If these muscles have active trigger points, strenuous activity may cause them to spasm.**

When using the technique with the strap wrapped around the ankle, use a long enough strap that the arms are comfortable. This will decrease the likelihood of aggravating muscles in the upper back, shoulder, and neck.

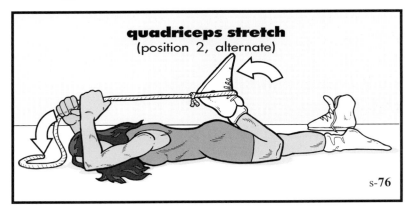

quadriceps stretch
(position 2, alternate)

s-76

223

Stretch

The stretch occurs as the ankle is pulled towards the head (see diagrams **s-75** and **s-76**).

Relaxation/Breathing

Using relaxation breathing techniques, focus on relaxing the neck, shoulder, hip, lower back, and thigh. Remember to inhale gently and exhale through the mouth, with a conscious puff of the lips. As the thigh muscles relax, pull the heel towards the buttocks, moving just enough to take up the slack of the relaxing muscles. Do not move beyond what will take up the slack. Slower motion and mindful relaxation will result in deeper levels of stretching.

Recovery

To recover from this stretch, simply relax the arm and lower the ankle.

⮞POSITION 3

The quadriceps can also be stretched lying on the back. This position requires the most flexibility of the three techniques. The heel of the thigh being stretched is placed as close to the buttocks as possible and is held by the hand on the same side (see diagram **s-77**).

Precautions

As the knee is lowered to the mat, the lower back will tend to arch. It is important to tighten the muscles in the front of the abdomen to keep the small of the back flat against the floor.

Stretch

The stretch is performed as the knee is lowered towards the floor by contracting the buttocks muscles (see diagram **s-77**). To help push the knee toward the floor, rest the heel of the opposite leg on the knee (not shown).

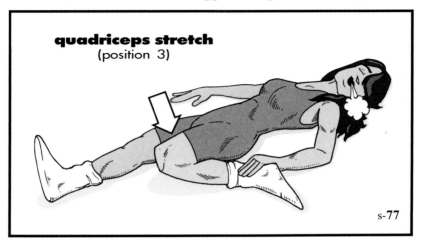

quadriceps stretch
(position 3)

s-77

Relaxation/Breathing

Using relaxation breathing techniques, focus on relaxing the lower back, buttocks, and thigh. Inhale gently and exhale through the mouth with a conscious puff of the lips. As the thigh muscles relax, lower the knee towards the floor. Do not move beyond what will take up the slack in the relaxing muscles. Slower motion and mindful relaxation will result in deeper levels of stretching.

Recovery

Allow the hip to flex and the knee to raise up, then straighten the knee.

ILIOPSOAS

The iliopsoas muscle crosses over the front of the hip joint and flexes the hip by moving the thigh forward and upward. It is stretched by extending the hip joint. There are two stretch positions described here for stretching this muscle. Use the position that allows the best relaxation and most frequent opportunities for stretching. The most important rule to follow with regard to positioning is that the iliopsoas muscle must be completely relaxed if stretching is to be effective and relatively comfortable.

These muscles are very important when treating lower back pain. Even if there are no thigh or groin pain symptoms, stretching these muscles should be considered whenever there is lower back pain.

Iliopsoas muscles get injured during running, lifting, and overstretching especially during play.

⮕POSITION 1

This stretch is most easily performed in a standing position. It is best to hold onto something on both sides of the body. The body weight will be supported by both hands and the foot placed to the front. The other foot will be placed behind the body, and the quadriceps muscle will be gently contracted to keep the knee straight, although perfectly straight is not important (see diagram **s-78**).

Precautions

The lower back should be stabilized by slightly tightening the muscles in the front of the abdomen. As the stretch progresses, do not allow the lower back and pelvis to tilt forward (sticking the buttocks out).

Stretch

The stretch is performed as the body is slowly moved forward and lowered toward the floor, allowing the hip joint to extend (see diagram **s-78**)

Relaxation/Breathing

Using relaxation breathing techniques, focus on relaxing the lower abdomen and the front of the hip. Remember to inhale gently and exhale

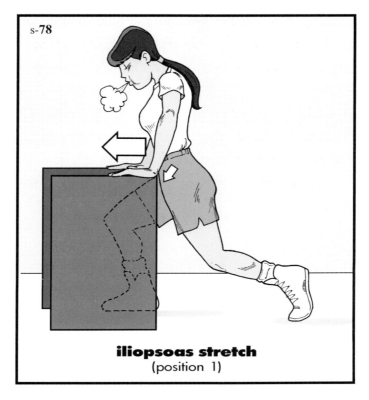

iliopsoas stretch
(position 1)

through the mouth, with a conscious puff of the lips. Keep the lower back upright, not leaning forward. As the hip muscles relax, hold the body weight with the forward foot and hands, and allow the body to go slowly forward and lower toward the floor. Do not move beyond what will take up the slack in the relaxing muscles. Slower motion and mindful relaxation will result in deeper levels of stretching.

Recovery

To recover from this stretch, push with the hands and the forward foot to raise up to a standing position.

▐▶POSITION 2

This stretch can also be performed low to the floor in a kneeling position. It is best to hold onto something on both sides of the body. The body weight will be stabilized by both hands and be supported by the bent knee and the foot placed to the front. The other foot will be placed behind the body (see diagram **s-79**).

Precautions

The lower back should be stabilized by slightly tightening the muscles in the front of the abdomen. As the stretch progresses, do not allow the lower back and pelvis to tilt forward (sticking the buttocks out). The **knee** of the backward leg **should be on a pillow** to protect the knee joint.

Stretch

The stretch is performed as the body is slowly moved forward and lowered

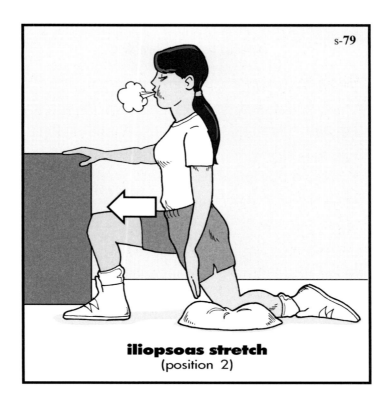

s-79

iliopsoas stretch
(position 2)

toward the floor, allowing the hip joint to extend (see diagram **s-79**).

Relaxation/Breathing

Using relaxation breathing techniques, focus on relaxing the lower abdomen and the front of the hip. Remember to inhale gently and exhale through the mouth, with a conscious puff of the lips. Keep the lower back upright, not leaning forward. As the hip muscles relax, stabilize the body weight with the forward foot and the hands, and allow the body to go slowly forward and lower toward the floor. Do not move beyond what will take up the slack in the relaxing muscles. Slower motion and mindful relaxation will result in deeper levels of stretching.

Recovery

To recover from this stretch, push with the hands and the forward foot to rock backward and raise up to a kneeling position.

HIP ADDUCTOR

The hip adductor muscles act primarily to bring the knees together. These muscles are very important when treating groin strain injuries, deep pelvic pain, inner thigh pain, and knee pain. They get injured during running and with the "foot-slipping splits."

⮕POSITION

This stretch is easiest to perform sitting on a flat cushion surface with the back supported. Bend the hips and knees, and pull the heels of the feet together and toward the groin (see diagram **s-80**). Then rest the hands on the knees.

Precautions

These muscles are fragile and do not tolerate a lot of force with stretching.

Overstretching can cause increased pain and make walking difficult. It is best to be gentle and not stretch much farther than the previous session.

Stretch

The stretch is performed as the hands gently push down and outward on the knees, spreading the thighs (see diagram **s-80**).

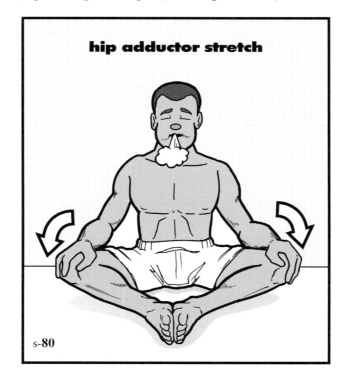

s-**80**

Relaxation/Breathing

Using relaxation breathing techniques, focus on relaxing the inner thighs and legs. Remember to inhale gently and exhale through the mouth with a conscious puff of the lips. As the hip muscles relax, allow the knees to fall toward the floor. Do not move beyond what will take up the slack in the relaxing muscles. Slower motion and mindful relaxation will result in deeper levels of stretching.

Recovery

To recover from this stretch, lift up the knees and move the feet to make the legs comfortable.

CALF

The muscles of the back of the calf include the gastrocnemius, soleus and tibialis posterior. Trigger points in these muscles are responsible for calf pain, calf cramps, and foot pain. The main muscles in the front of the calf (shin) are the tibialis anterior and toe extensors. Trigger points in these muscles are responsible for shin splints, pain over the top of the foot, and pain in the great toe.

GASTROCNEMIUS

The gastrocnemius muscle acts over both the ankle and knee joints, bending (flexing) the knee and pushing the foot down (plantar flexing the ankle). To stretch this muscle, the knee must be kept straight and the ankle/foot bent upwards (dorsiflexed).

These muscles are very important when treating knee, calf, ankle, and foot pain. They are also important when treating plantar fascitis and phantom limb pain after a below the knee amputation.

The gastrocnemius muscle gets injured during jumping, running, sudden starts, and walking long distances carrying extra weight.

➡️POSITION

This stretch is likely to be familiar because it is a common "runner's stretch." Position the body as in the diagram, with the knee straight for the leg being stretched (see diagram **s-81**). Alternatively, instead of bracing against a wall, the upper body can be supported with the hands placed on an object such as a dresser or kitchen counter (not shown).

Precautions

This muscle is very strong—accustomed to holding many times the weight of the body. It will not stretch effectively without relaxation. It is most helpful to have the hands support the upper body. Stretching this muscle on the stairs is discouraged because this is generally too much weight for fully relaxing the calf.

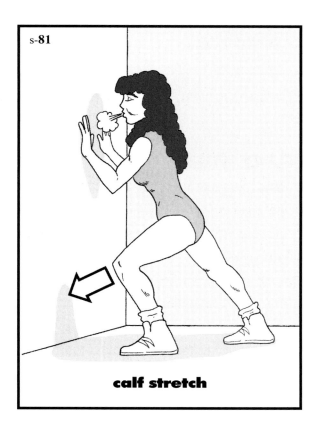

s-**81**

calf stretch

Stretch

The stretch occurs as the body is brought forward and the ankle bends upward (see diagram **s-81**).

Relaxation/Breathing

Using relaxation breathing techniques, focus on relaxing the back of the calf and gently keeping the knee straight. Once there is tension in the back of the calf, there will be little motion with each breath. Remember to inhale gently and exhale through the mouth with a conscious puff of the lips. As the calf muscles relax, allow the body to move forward, causing the ankle to further dorsiflex (bend upward). Do not move beyond what will take up the slack in the relaxing muscles. Slower motion and mindful relaxation will result in deeper levels of stretching.

Recovery

To recover from this stretch, push the body upright and stand on both feet.

SOLEUS AND TIBIALIS POSTERIOR

The soleus muscle acts only over the ankle joint and pushes the foot down. The tibialis posterior muscle supinates the foot and limits pronation when walking and running. In order to stretch these muscles the ankle must be bent upwards (dorsiflexed).

These muscles are important when treating calf pain, calf cramps, and foot pain, mostly in the heel and under the arch.

Jumping, running, sudden starts, and walking long distances carrying extra weight may cause injury to these muscles.

⮕POSITION

Position the body as in the diagram, with the knee bent and the ball of the foot propped up 2–4 inches (see diagram **s-82**).

Precautions

The soleus muscle is very strong—accustomed to holding many times the weight of the body. It will not stretch effectively without relaxation. If the foot is propped up against a wall, it is best to wear soft-soled shoes to protect the toe/foot joints.

Stretch

The stretch occurs as the knee is moved forward, bending the knee and the ankle at the same time (see diagram **s-82**).

Relaxation/Breathing

Using relaxation breathing techniques, focus on relaxing the back of

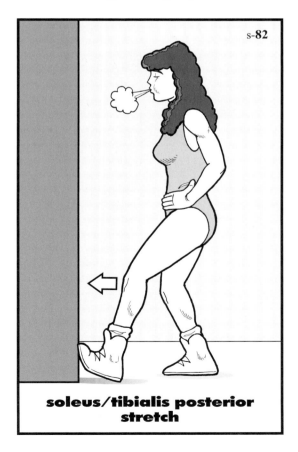

s-82

**soleus/tibialis posterior
stretch**

the calf. Once there is tension in the back of the calf, there will be little motion with each breath. Inhale gently and exhale through the mouth with a conscious puff of the lips. As the calf muscles relax, allow the knee to move forward, causing the ankle to further dorsiflex (bend upward). Do not move beyond what will take up the slack in the relaxing muscles. Slower motion and mindful relaxation will result in deeper levels of stretching.

Recovery

To recover from this stretch, contract the quadriceps (front of the thigh) and straighten the knee.

TIBIALIS ANTERIOR AND TOE EXTENSORS

The tibialis anterior acts over the front of the ankle joint. Contraction of the tibialis anterior bends the ankle to raise the foot. Contraction of the toe extensors straightens the toes. To stretch these muscles the ankle is plantar flexed (foot pushed downwards) and the toes are curled.

These muscles are very important when treating ankle, foot, and toe pain.

Tibialis anterior and toe extensor muscles are injured by walking and running, especially down hill with a firm heel strike.

➠POSITION

This muscle is most easily stretched in a seated position. Bring the left ankle up onto the right knee and hold the top of the left foot and the toes with the right hand (see diagrams **s-83** and **s-84**). For the other leg, do the opposite.

Precautions

This muscle is not very strong compared to the muscles of the back of

235

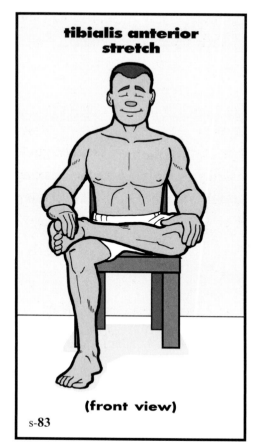

tibialis anterior stretch

(front view)

s-**83**

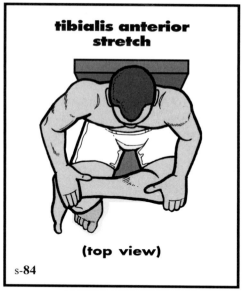

tibialis anterior stretch

(top view)

s-**84**

the calf. Relax well and do not apply much force with the hand. Try also to keep the shoulder and arm as relaxed as possible.

Stretch

Start the stretch with the hand placed over the top of the foot and gently pull toward the body. This will bend the ankle down, as in pushing on a pedal. After ankle motion stops,

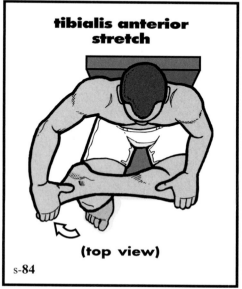

tibialis anterior stretch

(top view)

s-**84**

slowly slide the hand down over the tops of the toes, slowly bending the foot/ toe joints and pointing the toes back towards the body (see diagram **s-85**).

Relaxation/Breathing

Using relaxation breathing techniques, focus on relaxing the entire leg and foot being stretched. Remember to inhale gently and exhale through the mouth, with a conscious puff of the lips. As the leg muscles relax, guide the ankle and then the toes to stretch, taking up the slack in the relaxing muscles. Do not move beyond what will take up the slack of the relaxing muscles. Slower motion and mindful relaxation will result in deeper levels of stretching.

Recovery

To recover from this stretch, slowly let go of the toes and the foot.

PELVIC FLOOR

These muscles function with moving and holding body waste, and sexual functioning. Their pain patterns can be undiagnosed pelvic pain or misdiagnosed as interstitial cystitis. Stretching may involve internal myofascial release and is not discussed in this book. For this information, consult *Myofascial Pain and Dysfunction, The Trigger Point Manual*, volume 2, by Dr. Janet Travell and Dr. David Simons. Stretching the inner thighs, hamstrings, iliopsoas, and gluteal muscles may be helpful. Devin Starlanyl offers excellent suggestions in her book *Fibromyalgia and Myofascial Pain: A Survival Manual*, with Mary Ellen Copeland and Christopher R. Brown, 2001.

stretch

ADVANCED STRETCHING TECHNIQUE

Dr. David Simons, co-author of *Myofascial Pain and Dysfunction: The Trigger Point Manual* with Dr. Janet Travell, suggested that the "contract-relax" technique be included in this book. It is a simple thing and many people will find it helpful, especially when a muscle is not stretching well. Physical therapists consider this to be a "muscle energy" technique. It is usually performed by a therapist. Many of the stretches illustrated in this book can work well by adding this technique.

 Do not use this technique until you are familiar and comfortable with the basic stretching, breathing and relaxation principles described in the previous text.

Contract/Relax

During the process of stretching, pause and hold still in the position of stretch. During this pause, contract the muscle against resistance, with 30% power for 3–5 seconds. Then release the muscle and exhale at the same time, with a conscious puff of the lips. This relaxation after contraction enables more complete release of tension in the muscle being stretched.

Position/Timing

With all stretches, the time to start this technique is approximately 80% through the currently available stretch range of motion. Start the stretch and continue for a few to several breaths before starting the pause and contraction.

Precautions

Do not use more than partial muscle strength during the contract part of this technique. Overexertion may cause an increase in pain from trigger points in the muscle. It may also make other muscles more tired. This can cause an aggravation of pain symptoms if the muscle is fragile. Remember, it doesn't take much to aggravate the trigger points.

Stretch

Proceed through each basic stretch as described elsewhere in this book, adding the contract/relax technique in the middle.

Relaxation

After the contraction, perform the breathing and relaxation techniques as described in the *General Principles of Stretching* section (see page 123). The muscle will relax more and the body part may be moved to take up the slack.

This sequence may be repeated 3 times for any of the stretches.

Recovery

The recovery for each stretch is the same as that discussed earlier in the book.

stretch

picture index

picture index

Abdominal

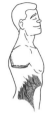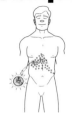
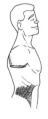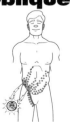
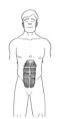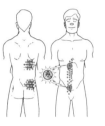
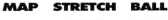
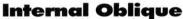
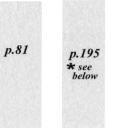
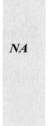
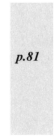
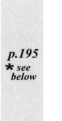
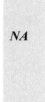
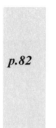
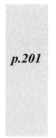
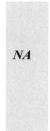

* muscle may not be specifically discussed in the **Ball** or **Stretch Chapters** but the techniques desribed are correct for this muscle/pain pattern

Arm

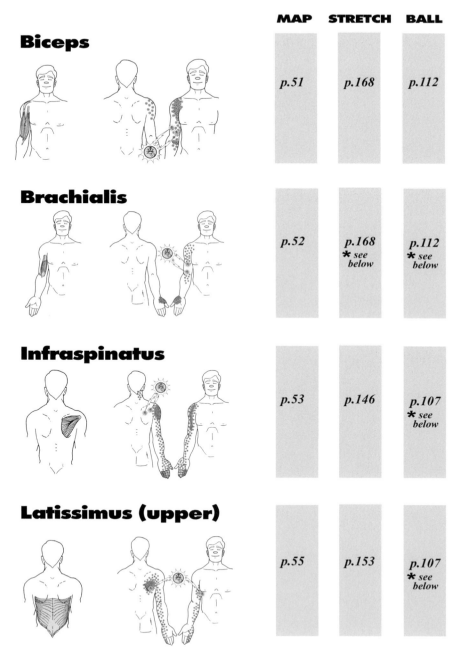

	MAP	STRETCH	BALL
Biceps	p.51	p.168	p.112
Brachialis	p.52	p.168 ✱ *see below*	p.112 ✱ *see below*
Infraspinatus	p.53	p.146	p.107 ✱ *see below*
Latissimus (upper)	p.55	p.153	p.107 ✱ *see below*

✱ muscle may not be specifically discussed in the **Ball** or **Stretch Chapters** but the techniques desribed are correct for this muscle/pain pattern

Arm

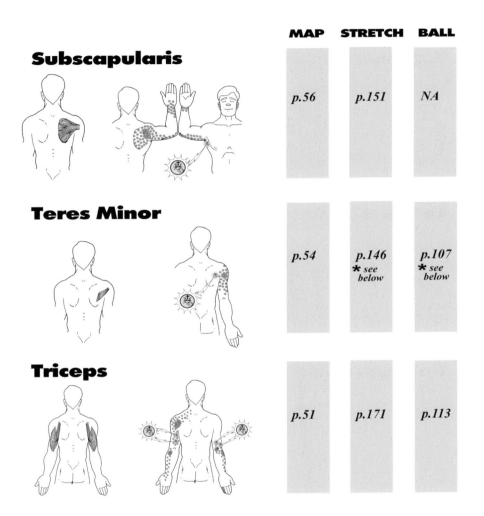

	MAP	STRETCH	BALL
Subscapularis	p.56	p.151	NA
Teres Minor	p.54	p.146 ***** *see below*	p.107 ***** *see below*
Triceps	p.51	p.171	p.113

* muscle may not be specifically discussed in the **Ball** or **Stretch Chapters**
but the techniques desribed are correct for this muscle/pain pattern

Back (lower)

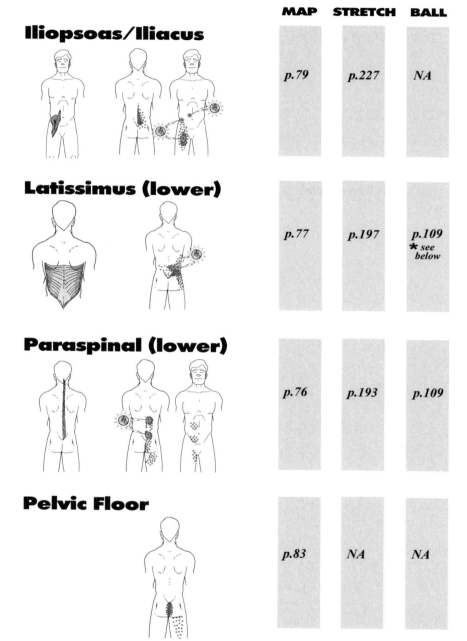

	MAP	STRETCH	BALL
Iliopsoas/Iliacus	p.79	p.227	NA
Latissimus (lower)	p.77	p.197	p.109 ✱ see below
Paraspinal (lower)	p.76	p.193	p.109
Pelvic Floor	p.83	NA	NA

✱ muscle may not be specifically discussed in the **Ball** or **Stretch Chapters** but the techniques desribed are correct for this muscle/pain pattern

Back (lower)

Quadratus Lumborum

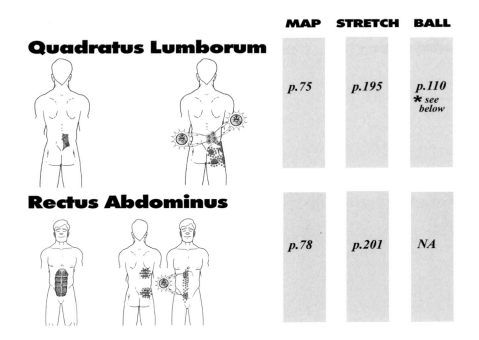

	MAP	STRETCH	BALL
Quadratus Lumborum	*p.75*	*p.195*	*p.110* ***** *see below*
Rectus Abdominus	*p.78*	*p.201*	NA

Rectus Abdominus

Back (upper)

Infraspinatus

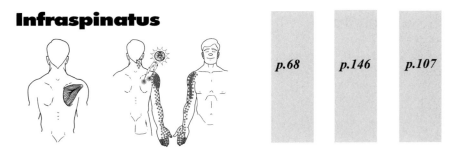

	MAP	STRETCH	BALL
Infraspinatus	*p.68*	*p.146*	*p.107*

* muscle may not be specifically discussed in the **Ball** or **Stretch Chapters** but the techniques desribed are correct for this muscle/pain pattern

Back (upper)

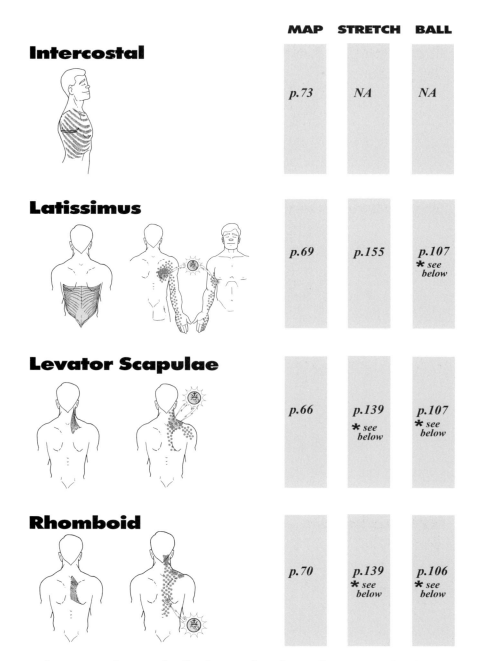

	MAP	STRETCH	BALL
Intercostal	p.73	NA	NA
Latissimus	p.69	p.155	p.107 * see below
Levator Scapulae	p.66	p.139 * see below	p.107 * see below
Rhomboid	p.70	p.139 * see below	p.106 * see below

* muscle may not be specifically discussed in the **Ball** or **Stretch Chapters**
but the techniques desribed are correct for this muscle/pain pattern

Back (upper)

	MAP	STRETCH	BALL
Serratus Posterior Superior	*p.71*	*p.139* ✻ *see below*	*p.108* ✻ *see below*
Supraspinatus	*p.67*	*p.137* ✻ *see below*	*p.108* ✻ *see below*
Paraspinal (upper)	*p.72*	*p.193* ✻ *see below*	*p.106* ✻ *see below*
Trapezius (mid/ lower)	*p.73*	*p.193* ✻ *see below*	*p.106* ✻ *see below*

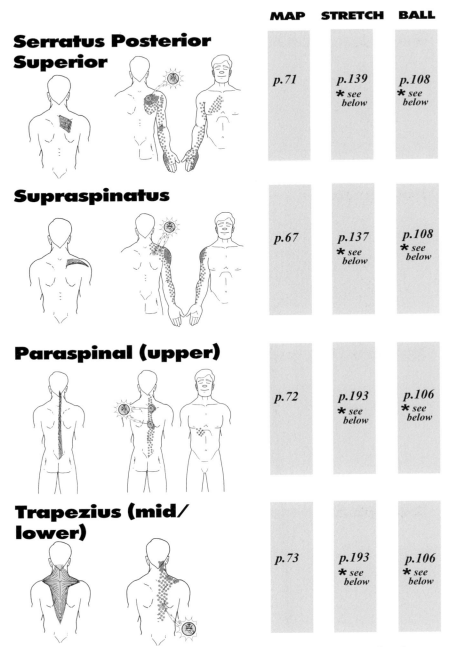

✱ muscle may not be specifically discussed in the **Ball** or **Stretch Chapters** but the techniques desribed are correct for this muscle/pain pattern

Calf and Lower Leg

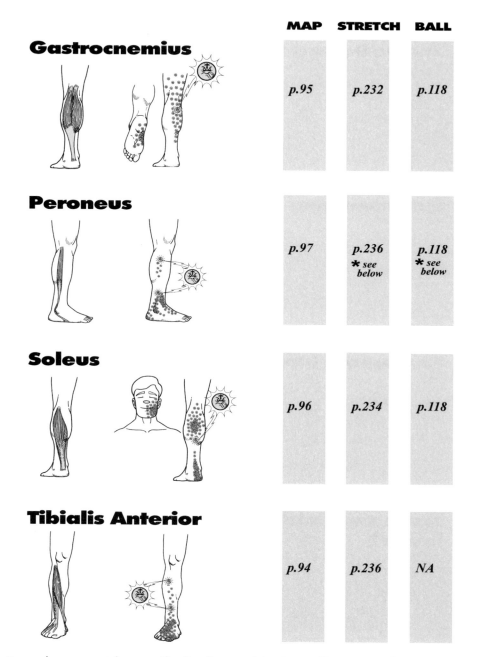

	MAP	STRETCH	BALL
Gastrocnemius	*p.95*	*p.232*	*p.118*
Peroneus	*p.97*	*p.236* ✱ *see below*	*p.118* ✱ *see below*
Soleus	*p.96*	*p.234*	*p.118*
Tibialis Anterior	*p.94*	*p.236*	*NA*

✱ muscle may not be specifically discussed in the **Ball** or **Stretch Chapters** but the techniques desribed are correct for this muscle/pain pattern

Calf and Lower Leg

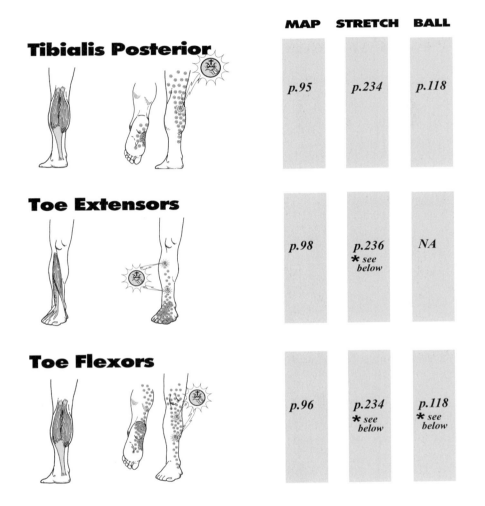

	MAP	STRETCH	BALL
Tibialis Posterior	p.95	p.234	p.118
Toe Extensors	p.98	p.236 * see below	NA
Toe Flexors	p.96	p.234 * see below	p.118 * see below

* muscle may not be specifically discussed in the **Ball** or **Stretch Chapters**
but the techniques desribed are correct for this muscle/pain pattern

pict index

Elbow and Wrist

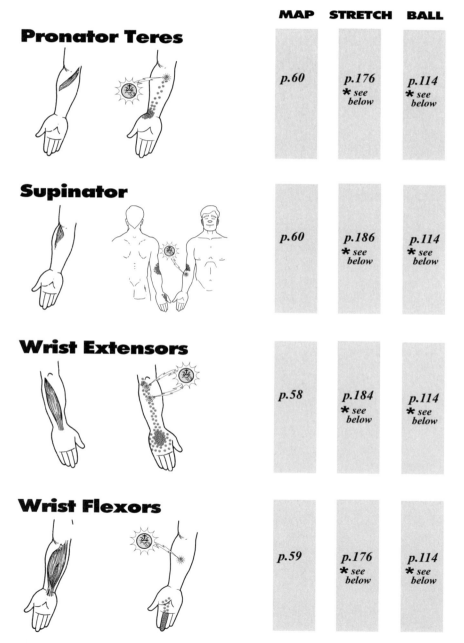

	MAP	STRETCH	BALL
Pronator Teres	p.60	p.176 * see below	p.114 * see below
Supinator	p.60	p.186 * see below	p.114 * see below
Wrist Extensors	p.58	p.184 * see below	p.114 * see below
Wrist Flexors	p.59	p.176 * see below	p.114 * see below

* muscle may not be specifically discussed in the **Ball** or **Stretch Chapters**
but the techniques desribed are correct for this muscle/pain pattern

Foot

	MAP	STRETCH	BALL
Foot (bottom)	*p.99*	*p.234* ✱ *see below*	*p.119*
Foot (top)	*p.99*	*p.236* ✱ *see below*	*NA*

Forearm

	MAP	STRETCH	BALL
Palmaris Longus	*p.62*	*p.176*	*p.114* ✱ *see below*

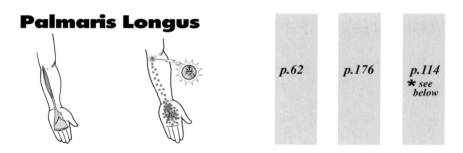

✱ muscle may not be specifically discussed in the **Ball** or **Stretch Chapters** but the techniques desribed are correct for this muscle/pain pattern

Hand and Finger

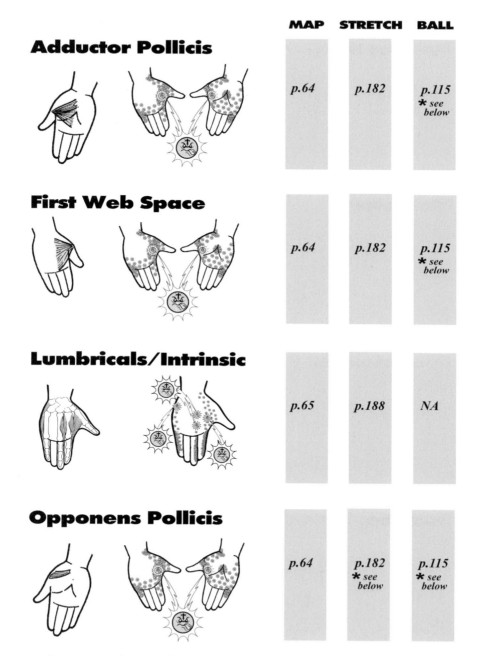

	MAP	STRETCH	BALL
Adductor Pollicis	p.64	p.182	p.115 ** see below*
First Web Space	p.64	p.182	p.115 ** see below*
Lumbricals/Intrinsic	p.65	p.188	NA
Opponens Pollicis	p.64	p.182 ** see below*	p.115 ** see below*

* muscle may not be specifically discussed in the **Ball** or **Stretch Chapters**
but the techniques desribed are correct for this muscle/pain pattern

Head and Neck

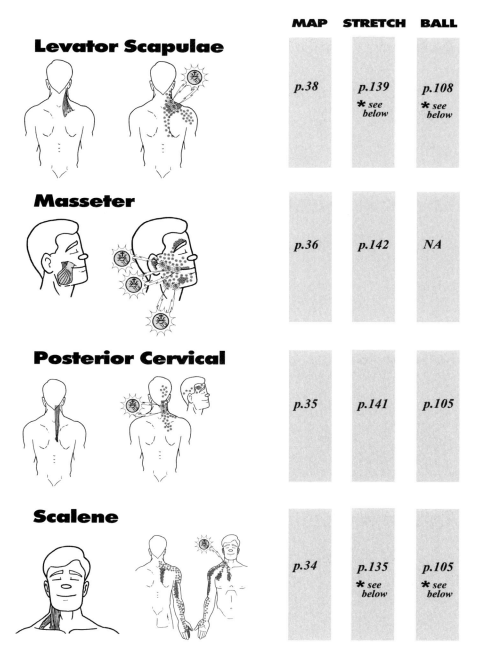

	MAP	STRETCH	BALL
Levator Scapulae	p.38	p.139 *see below	p.108 *see below
Masseter	p.36	p.142	NA
Posterior Cervical	p.35	p.141	p.105
Scalene	p.34	p.135 *see below	p.105 *see below

✱ muscle may not be specifically discussed in the **Ball** or **Stretch Chapters**
but the techniques desribed are correct for this muscle/pain pattern

Head and Neck

	MAP	STRETCH	BALL
Soleus 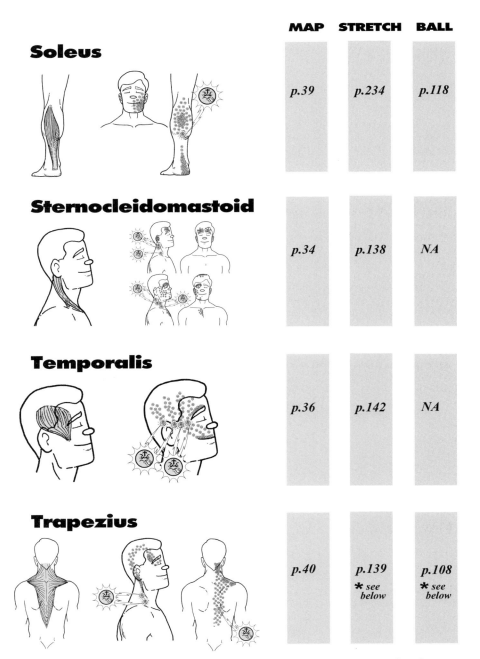	*p.39*	*p.234*	*p.118*
Sternocleidomastoid	*p.34*	*p.138*	*NA*
Temporalis	*p.36*	*p.142*	*NA*
Trapezius	*p.40*	*p.139* ** see below*	*p.108* ** see below*

✱ muscle may not be specifically discussed in the **Ball** or **Stretch Chapters**
but the techniques desribed are correct for this muscle/pain pattern

254

Hip and Buttocks

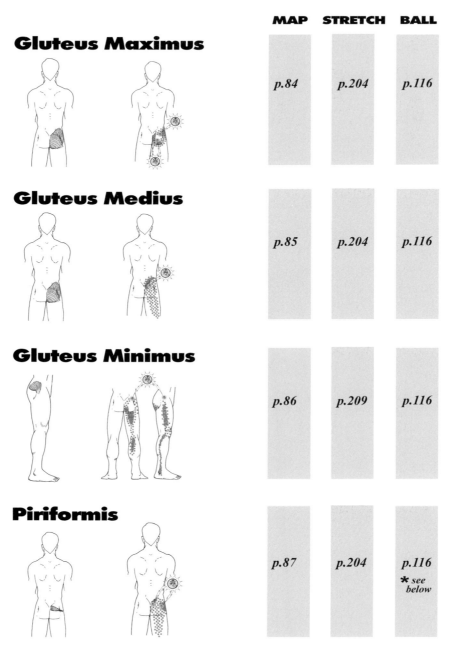

	MAP	STRETCH	BALL
Gluteus Maximus	p.84	p.204	p.116
Gluteus Medius	p.85	p.204	p.116
Gluteus Minimus	p.86	p.209	p.116
Piriformis	p.87	p.204	p.116 * *see below*

✻ muscle may not be specifically discussed in the **Ball** or **Stretch Chapters** but the techniques desribed are correct for this muscle/pain pattern

Hip and Buttocks

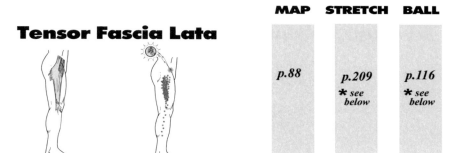

Tensor Fascia Lata

MAP	STRETCH	BALL
p.88	p.209 *see below	p.116 *see below

Shoulder

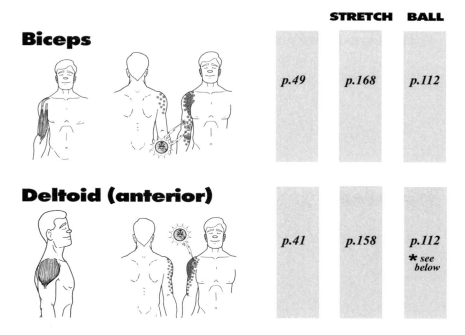

Biceps

	STRETCH	BALL
p.49	p.168	p.112

Deltoid (anterior)

	STRETCH	BALL
p.41	p.158	p.112 *see below

✱ muscle may not be specifically discussed in the **Ball** or **Stretch Chapters** but the techniques desribed are correct for this muscle/pain pattern

Shoulder

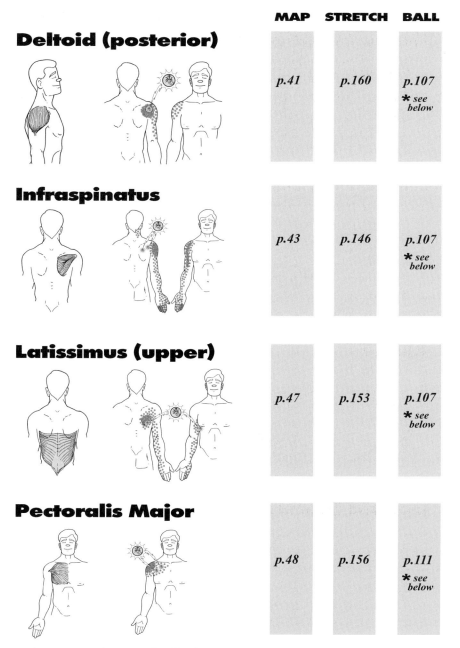

	MAP	STRETCH	BALL
Deltoid (posterior)	p.41	p.160	p.107 **✳** see below
Infraspinatus	p.43	p.146	p.107 **✳** see below
Latissimus (upper)	p.47	p.153	p.107 **✳** see below
Pectoralis Major	p.48	p.156	p.111 **✳** see below

✳ muscle may not be specifically discussed in the **Ball** or **Stretch Chapters** but the techniques desribed are correct for this muscle/pain pattern

Shoulder

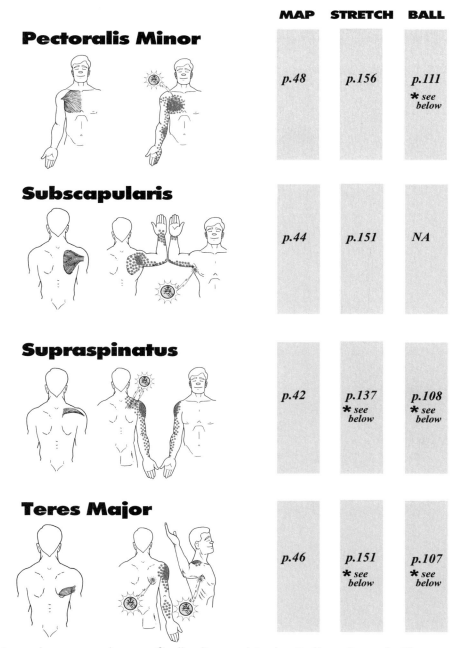

	MAP	STRETCH	BALL
Pectoralis Minor	p.48	p.156	p.111 * see below
Subscapularis	p.44	p.151	NA
Supraspinatus	p.42	p.137 * see below	p.108 * see below
Teres Major	p.46	p.151 * see below	p.107 * see below

* muscle may not be specifically discussed in the **Ball** or **Stretch Chapters** but the techniques desribed are correct for this muscle/pain pattern

Shoulder

	MAP	STRETCH	BALL
Teres Minor	p.45	p.146 *see below	p.107 *see below
Trapezius	p.40	p.139 *see below	p.106 *see below
Triceps	p.49	p.172	p.113

* muscle may not be specifically discussed in the **Ball** or **Stretch Chapters** but the techniques desribed are correct for this muscle/pain pattern

Thigh

	MAP	STRETCH	BALL
Hamstrings	p.93	p.212	p.117 ** see below*
Hip Adductor	p.92	p.230	NA
Quadriceps	p.90	p.221	NA

* muscle may not be specifically discussed in the **Ball** or **Stretch Chapters** but the techniques desribed are correct for this muscle/pain pattern

Thigh

	MAP	STRETCH	BALL

Sartorius

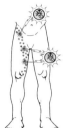 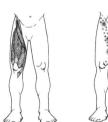 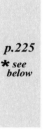 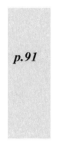 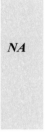

| | *p.91* | *p.225*
✱ see below | *NA* |

Tensor Fascia Lata

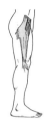 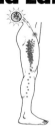 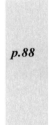 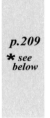 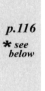

| | *p.88* | *p.209*
✱ see below | *p.116*
✱ see below |

✱ muscle may not be specifically discussed in the **Ball** or **Stretch Chapters** but the techniques desribed are correct for this muscle/pain pattern

pict index

index

index

shoulder pain, 39, 48–51
stretching, 167–170
Bleeding. See Bruise; Contusion
Brachialis muscle, arm pain, 52
Brachioradialis, 57
Breathing, 123–124
  diaphragmatic, 124
  technique for, 125–126
    as tool to relax, 122
  See also Stretching
Brown, Christopher R., 237
Bruise, 26–27
Bunion pain, 100
Bursitis, 5, 10, 88
Buttock/hamstring massage, 116–117
Buttocks pain. See Hip and buttocks pain

C

Calf, stretching, 231–237
  gastrocnemius, 231–233
  soleus and tibialis posterior, 233–235
  tibialis anterior and toe extensors,
    235–237
Calf and lower leg pain, 94–98
  gastrocnemius, tibialis posterior, and
    soleus, 95–96
  peroneus (longus, brevis, tertius), 97
  tibialis anterior and toe extensors, 94–95
  toe extensors, 97–98
  toe flexors, 96
Carpal tunnel syndrome (CTS), 5, 47
  and forearm pain, 61
  biceps and, 48–50
  causes of, 165–167
  massage techniques for, 112
  new theory, 166
  new treatment, 166–167
  old theory, 165
  stretching, 174–179
  traditional treatment, 165–166
Chest massage, 110–111
Chest pain, 46–48
  See also Pleurisy
Chest stretches. See Upper back, shoulder,

and chest stretches
Chronic pain
  myofascial pain model for, 16–19
  treatment of myofascial pain to diminish,
    20–23
  See also Myofascial pain; Pain
Contract-relax techniques, 238–239
Contusion, 26–27
Conventional medical training, 8
Copeland, Mary Ellen, 237
Cortisone, 165–166
CTS. See Carpal tunnel syndrome (CTS)

D

Deltoid
  pain, 39, 41–42
  stretching, 157–163
Depressed middle aged woman model, 14
Depression, pain from, 10
Diaphragmatic breathing, 124
Dorsiflexors, 57–58

E

Elbow and wrist pain, 57–61
  pronator teres, 60–61
  supinator, 59–60
  wrist extensors (dorsiflexors), 57–58
  wrist flexors (palmar flexors), 58–59
Ergonomic factors, for myofascial
  pain syndrome, 19–20
Ethyl Chloride. See Vapocoolant spray
Exercise, stretching before and after,
  131–132
Extensor carpi radialis brevis, 57
Extensor carpi radialis longus, 57
Extensor carpi ulnaris, 57
External obliques
  pain, 81–82
Extremities (upper)
  biceps (massage), 112
  biceps (stretch), 167–170
  carpal tunnel syndrome (CTS), 164–167
  forearm (carpal tunnel syndrome,
    golfer's elbow), 174–179

notes

notes

273

"As a Rolfer, many clients I see are searching for a way out of pain. Because of the complexity of the body, it can be a challenge for people to know precisely which muscles cause their pain and/or how to improve their symptoms. Dr. Blatman has skillfully blended his medical knowledge and training with humor and simplicity to create an exemplary tool that anyone can utilize with ease. The Winners' Guide to Pain Relief is packed with practical and effective information that helps us learn more about the body, find ways to alleviate pain, and thereby accelerate the recovery process."

Wanda L Sucher, LMT, KDK
Advanced Certified Rolfer
Certified Yoga Instructor
Thai Yoga Therapist
Director of Lifepath Center of the Healing Arts

"*The Art of Body Maintenance: Winners' Guide to Pain Relief* is truly a remarkable book that will be a boon to pain patients and practitioners alike. Dr. Blatman explains the main causes of patients' pain and describes step-by-step how to stop pain and keep it from coming back. He does so in plain, clear, precise language that is rare for pain-relief experts. On practically every page, artist Brad Ekvall's drawings beautifully illustrate what Dr. Blatman's words clearly convey, making the book as understandable and useful as a self-help guide can possible be. Both pain patients and pain practitioners are certain to treasure this book, as I do, and make it tread-bare from regular use."

John C Lowe, MA, DC
Author of *The Metabolic Treatment of Fibromyalgia Your Guide to Metabolic Health*